LOCAL ANALGESIA IN DENTISTRY

LOCAL ANALGESIA IN DENTISTRY

BY

D. H. ROBERTS FDS RCS

Honorary Lecturer, Department of Conservative Dentistry, Institute of Dental Surgery, Eastman Dental Hospital, London

AND

J. H. SOWRAY BDS, FRCS, FDS RCS

Professor and Head of Department of Oral and Maxillo-facial Surgery, King's College Hospital, London

WITH A FOREWORD BY

PROFESSOR SIR ROBERT BRADLAW

Third Edition

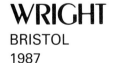

WRIGHT

BRISTOL

1987

Published under the Wright imprint by
IOP Publishing Limited
Techno House, Redcliffe Way, Bristol BS1 6NX

First edition, 1970
Reprinted, 1976
Second edition, 1979
Reprinted, 1983
Third edition, 1987
Italian edition, 1972
Japanese edition, 1976
Spanish edition, 1982

British Library Cataloguing in Publication Data
Roberts, D.H. (Derek Harry)
  Local analgesia in dentistry.—3rd ed.
  1. Anesthesia in dentistry   2. Local anaesthesia
  I. Title   II. Sowray, J.H.
  617′.9676   RK510

ISBN 0 7236 0954 3

Origination by
EJS Chemical Composition, Midsomer Norton, Bath BA3 4BQ

Printed in Great Britain by
The Bath Press, Lower Bristol Road, Bath BA2 3BL

PREFACE

The purpose of this new edition remains unchanged in that it seeks to be an up-to-date guide to dental local analgesia for students and practitioners. We have described the latest advances, but hope that our emphasis has remained on the practical aspects of the subject.

We are most grateful for the helpful suggestions received from many colleagues and, in addition to those previously acknowledged, we would particularly like to record our thanks to Dr E. A. Fagan, Mr M. G. D. Kelleher, Mr M. Ljungberg, Dr Ian Martin, Dr Caroline Pankhurst, Dr Stelios Pateromichelakis, Dr José Ponte, Professor J. P. Rood, Mr Keith Watson and Dr S. R. Watt-Smith. Mrs Joan Weinstock and Miss Fiona Murray gave valuable help with the typescript.

March 1987
D. H. R.
J. H. S.

PREFACE TO THE FIRST EDITION

The commonest and safest method of preventing pain during dental treatment is the use of local analgesia. In recent years there have been considerable advances both in the drugs used and in the equipment for their administration. At the same time, modern medical therapy has introduced problems which may have to be carefully considered when a patient's fitness for local analgesia is assessed. The purpose of this book is to discuss these matters and to provide a practical guide to the subject.

The sections on techniques, precautions and instruments have been expanded to lay emphasis on the safest methods of achieving local analgesia. Although prilocaine and lignocaine are the most commonly used preparations in the UK, others have been mentioned to show how the search for the ideal local analgesic has progressed.

April 1970
D. H. R.
J. H. S.

ACKNOWLEDGEMENTS

Our introduction to local analgesia—or local anaesthesia as it used to be termed—was provided by Mr B. W. Fickling at the Royal Dental Hospital and we are indebted to him for his teaching, which has undoubtedly influenced us in our writing.

This book could not have been written without the generous help and advice of many colleagues, and among those we should particularly like to thank are Mr F. Allott of the Medical Protection Society; Dr R. C. Bret Day; Mr S. L. Drummond-Jackson and his colleagues of the Society for the Advancement of Anaesthesia in Dentistry; Dr P. T. Flute; Dr G. H. Forman; Dr W. Fraser-Moodie; Mr A. R. Halder; Dr M. Harris; Mr F. J. Harty; Dr C. D. T. James; Mr A. Kinghorn; Mr L. J. Leggett; Dr J. F. Lockwood; Professor H. McIlwain; Dr I. P. Priban; photogenic Miss B. S. Ray; Dr D. A. Pyke; Mr A. H. Rowe of the Medical Defence Union; Professor M. J. H. Smith; and Mr G. F. Tinsley.

We owe special debts of gratitude to Dr A. H. Galley and Dr Victor Goldman for their expert help with the sections on pharmacology, pre-medication, and allied topics; to Professor H. C. Killey for information regarding his researches on vasoconstrictors; and to Professor G. R. Seward and Dr R. Haskell for their helpful comments and criticisms of the text. Dr F. Stansfield kindly devoted a lot of time in advising on the anatomy chapter. Mr C. L. M. Brown and his colleagues at the Pharmaceutical Manufacturing Company generously showed us the process of producing local analgesics and Mr Roger Hickson of Messrs Cottrell and Company was extremely helpful with his technical knowledge of instruments.

The majority of the illustrations and photographs were the artistic work of Miss Jennifer Middleton and Mr J. Morgan, respectively. Mrs Angela Birbeck, Mr E. W. Blewett, Mrs Margaret Cooper, Mr P. Kertesz and Mr N. Pearson also kindly helped in this field. The typescript was very ably prepared by Mrs Maria Harrison, Mrs P. Mouncer and Mrs P. Procter.

CONTENTS

FOREWORD TO THE FIRST EDITION

By SIR ROBERT BRADLAW CBE

Professor of Oral Medicine, University of London
Honorary Professor of Dental Pathology,
Royal College of Surgeons of England

I am very glad to contribute a brief foreword to this admirable book, not only because of the importance of its subject but for its eminently sensible and essentially practical approach. Written attractively with commend-able lucidity and directness, it affords a succinct account of what is currently known of analgesia—its mechanism, technique, pharmacology, instrumentarium and application.

For the best of reasons, anaesthesia and analgesia have long been of special interest to both clinician and patient. Ever since the seventeenth century, when the Royal Society became interested in the use of drugs, especially narcotics, for the relief of pain, considerable thought and effort have been devoted to the better understanding of their rationale.

We have learnt much in consequence as to the mode of action, appli-cation and of the physiological response of the tissues. It might be thought that this would make the task of the clinician simpler, but this is not the case, for concurrently with our better understanding of pharmacological principles and advances in technique we have recognized new potential hazards and the possibility of complications not known to an earlier generation.

The management of patients with cardiovascular lesions, for example, the risks inherent in sickle-cell anaemia, the effects of steroid therapy and other iatrogenic manifestations impose a far greater clinical and legal responsibility on the dental surgeon than hitherto.

This comprehensive and authoritative text should be read by specialist and general practitioners alike; there are few of us who would not find it interesting and helpful. Its usefulness is further enhanced by well-chosen references for further reading, a list of trade and alternative names for analgesic drugs and, topically, a metric conversion table.

Chapter 1

DEVELOPMENT OF LOCAL ANALGESIA

The use of local analgesia followed the development of the hypodermic syringe with its hollow needle (*Figs.* 1.1, 1.2). In 1827 von Neuner produced one which was designed for injecting drugs used in ophthalmic veterinary work. In 1841 an American, Zophar Jayne, patented another type which had a pointed needle, but its insertion into the tissues was facilitated by first incising the skin with a lancet. Some 3 years later Francis Rynd of Dublin started administering drugs subcutaneously using an elaborate stylet, the solution being forced into the tissues by means of gravity (*Fig.* 1.3). Thus, although

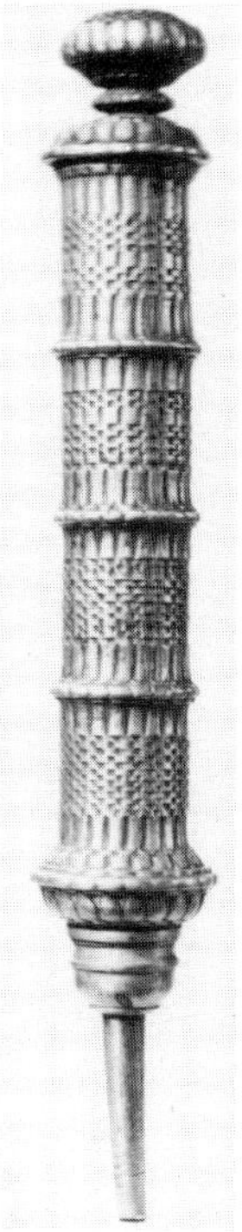

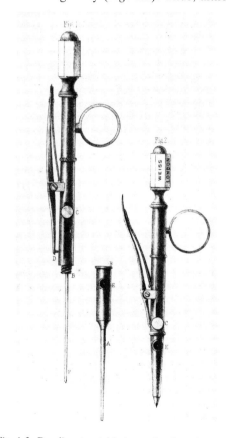

Fig. 1.1 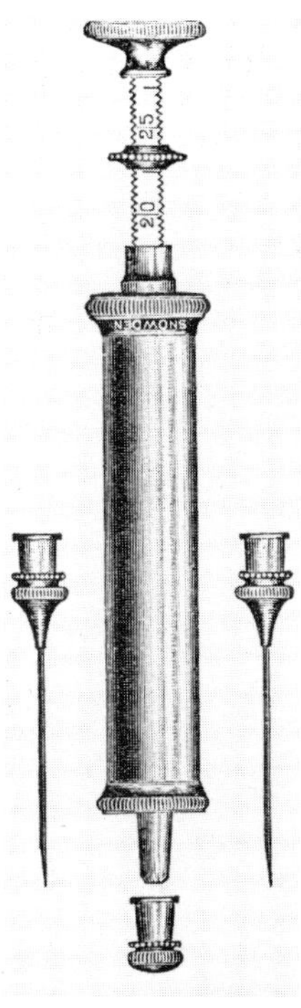   Fig. 1.2

Fig. 1.1. Seventeenth-century French syringe of the type from which the hypodermic syringe was developed. Wellcome Historical Medical Museum No. R3655/1936. (*Figs.* 1.1–1.8 are reproduced by courtesy of the Wellcome Trustees.)

Fig. 1.2. An early German silver hypodermic syringe illustrated in *A Manual of Hypodermatic Medication,* by R. Bartholow, 1882, 4th ed. Philadelphia, Lippincott.

Fig. 1.3. Rynd's retractable trocar for the subcutaneous injection of liquids. (From *Dublin Quarterly Journal of Medical Science,* 1861, **32**, 13.)

this was not strictly a hypodermic syringe, it was very similar in action.

A hypodermic syringe of all-metal construction was invented in 1853 by a French veterinary surgeon, Charles Gabriel Pravaz (*Figs.* 1.4, 1.5). It was a well-designed instrument with

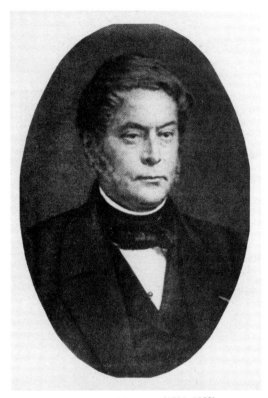

Fig. 1.4. Charles Gabriel Pravaz (1791–1853).

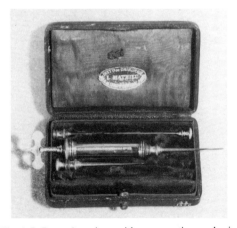

Fig. 1.5. Pravaz's syringe with screw action and minute trocars and cannula. Wellcome Historical Medical Museum No. 32/1950.

a screw piston rod which enabled precise doses to be given accurately, but, although it was used for administering some drugs, it was not employed to obtain local analgesia. At about the same time Alexander Wood, of Edinburgh, was using a hypodermic syringe for the injection of opiates subcutaneously for the relief of neuralgia. His syringe was made of glass and metal and was a modification of the Ferguson type (*Fig.* 1.6).

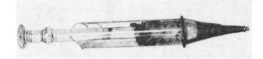

Fig. 1.6. The original hypodermic syringe used by Alexander Wood. Museum of the Royal College of Surgeons of Edinburgh. (From Comrie, J. D. (1932), *History of Scottish Medicine,* 2nd ed., vol. II. London, Baillière, Tindall and Cox, p. 614.)

For centuries the natives of Bolivia and Peru had been addicted to coca, a mixture of dried leaves containing cocaine which they used because of its exhilarating effect, their custom being to extract the cocaine by chewing the coca with lime which masked the bitter taste. In 1855 a French chemist, Gaedcke, obtained a crude extract of cocaine from the South American plant *Erythroxylum coca* and 5 years later pure cocaine was isolated by Albert Niemann while working in Frederick Wohler's laboratory, following which extensive studies were made of its pharmacological actions. In 1880 a Russian surgeon, Vasilius von Anrep, reported on the numbing action of cocaine on mucous membranes, and in 1884 Carl Köller (*Fig.* 1.7), a colleague of the Austrian psychoanalyst Sigmund Freud, wrote a paper describing its analgesic action on the eye. After Freud received this paper he nicknamed his colleague Coca Köller, possibly being inspired by the beverage which had been created by an American pharmacist, John S. Pemberton, at about that time. Freud himself had previously considered the use of cocaine for treating eye diseases, but, as D. R. Laurence comments, 'appreciating that sex was of greater importance than surgery', he had gone on holiday with his fiancée, thus leaving Köller to discover the anaesthetic properties of cocaine which became so valuable in clinical ophthalmology.

In November 1884, exactly 40 years after

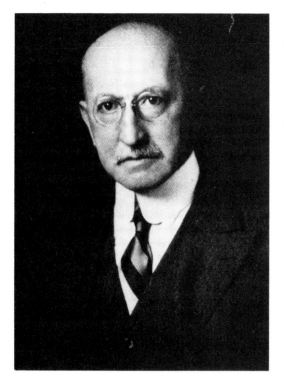

Fig. 1.7. Carl Köller (1857–1944).

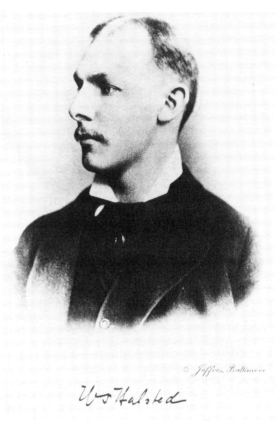

Fig. 1.8. William Stewart Halsted (1852–1922). (From Halsted's *Surgical Papers*, 1924. Baltimore, Johns Hopkins.)

nitrous oxide was first used for general anaesthesia, William Halsted (*Fig.* 1.8), at the Bellevue Hospital, New York City, carried out the first blocking of the mandibular nerve by injecting 4 per cent cocaine intraorally. His patients were his first assistant, Dr Richard John Hall, and a medical student, Mr Locke. Dr Hall reported, in a letter published in the *New York Medical Journal* of 6 December 1884, that he had also had painless dental treatment of his upper left incisor tooth after being given an infraorbital nerve block. Halsted, who was a brilliant surgeon and pioneered surgical treatment of carcinoma of the breast, unfortunately became addicted to cocaine, as did Dr Hall. Following this early work, cocaine became widely used for local analgesia and thus its shortcomings and dangers soon became apparent. This stimulated further research to discover other drugs which did not have its disadvantages and in 1904 a German chemist, Alfred Einhorn, synthesized procaine, which for many years remained the most commonly used local analgesic.

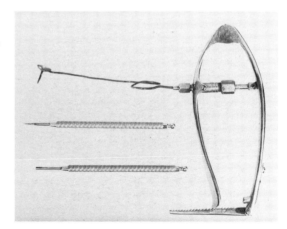

Fig. 1.9. The Wilcox–Jewel 'obtunder' type of high-pressure syringe, 1904.

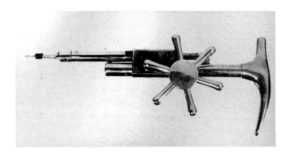

Fig. 1.10. Thew's capstan pattern high-pressure syringe, 1912.

In 1904 a high-pressure syringe was introduced, known as the Wilcox–Jewel 'obtunder', powered by a leaf spring (*Fig*. 1.9). Another type of high-pressure syringe was produced by the Dental Manufacturing Company in 1912 to a design credited to Dr Thew. This syringe utilized a capstan (*Fig*. 1.10).

In 1917 Harvey S. Cook devised the cartridge system for loading syringes and this considerably simplified the chair-side process of preparation and sterilization of the analgesic drug.

In 1943 a Swedish chemist, Nils Löfgren, synthesized lignocaine and 5 years later this product was marketed. This local analgesic drug is still by far the most commonly used at the present time, although newer products such as prilocaine, with felypressin as a vasoconstrictor, are now available.

The more recent developments in local analgesia include the commoner use of the intra-periodontal or intraligamentary injection for conservation, increased availability of pre-sterilized equipment, improvements in the design of jet injectors, the removal of the preservatives from some local anaesthetic solutions because of their adverse reactions, and research into reversing the effects of local anaesthetics. These and other changes will be discussed in the later chapters.

REFERENCES AND FURTHER READING

Laurence D. R. (1969) *Clinical Pharmacology*, 3rd ed. London, Churchill, p. 206.
McAuley J. E. (1966) The early development of local anaesthesia. *Br. Dent. J.* **121,** 139.
Matas R. (1952) The story of the discovery of dental anaesthesia by nerve blocking. *Surgery* **32,** 530.

Chapter 2

METHODS OF CONTROLLING DENTAL PAIN

Analgesia is a condition in which pain cannot be appreciated but the patient is aware of what is happening. 'General analgesia' means the loss of the sensation of pain throughout the body and can be induced with drugs such as nitrous oxide or Trilene (trichloroethylene), which may be used during labour. 'Local analgesia' means the loss of the sensation of pain in a limited region and can be induced by surface application or infiltration, and regional injection of drugs.

Anaesthesia means the complete loss of all sensation including that of pain, although this word is sometimes inaccurately used to describe the loss of only tactile sensation. 'General anaesthesia' is a condition in which the patient does not react to any stimuli, including pain, and also does not have any memory of what has been happening, which implies that the patient has been unconscious. The term 'local anaesthesia' means that a potent drug has been used to produce the temporary loss of all modalities of sensation in a limited region of the body.

Usually in dentistry we are attempting to obtain analgesia because we wish to prevent pain. Sometimes we will also achieve anaesthesia and this may be desirable, although theoretically surplus to our requirements, as it should not matter whether our patient is aware of tactile sensation or not. However, some patients, particularly those of low intelligence, have difficulty in appreciating the differences between touch or pressure and actual pain and this is sometimes responsible for apparent failures in local analgesia.

Local analgesia is obtained most commonly by placing a drug called an analgesic near the sensory nerves so as to temporarily prevent the conduction of pain impulses to the brain. This deposition is usually carried out by injecting a solution into the tissues.

In dental surgery local analgesia of the teeth is obtained in two basic ways. It may be achieved by *infiltration analgesia,* which is the deposition of an analgesic solution close to the apex of the tooth so that it can diffuse to reach the nerves entering the apical foramina. The second technique, known as *regional analgesia,* is to block the passage of pain impulses by depositing analgesic close to a nerve trunk, thus cutting off the sensory innervation to the region it supplies. This injection is normally at a site where the nerve is unprotected by bone and therefore readily accessible to the solution.

DENTAL USES OF LOCAL ANALGESIA

1. Elimination of pain during treatment

This is the most common use of local analgesia in dental surgery. By its employment the dental surgeon is able to carry out painlessly routine treatment such as the extraction or conservation of teeth. Similarly, minor oral surgery for the removal of small cysts and tumours, periodontal surgery, and, in special circumstances, quite major operations may be performed. For example, when a dental surgeon is on active service in war zones or working in remote parts of the world, he may have to treat severe jaw injuries under local analgesia because the more elaborate facilities required for working under general anaesthesia are not available.

Allied to the use of local analgesia for eliminating pain during treatment is its use to assist in relaxing patients. Some people are difficult to treat, not because the dental surgeon is hurting them, but because they think that he may be about to do so. If a local analgesic drug has been administered then the patient knows that whatever the dental surgeon does during the treatment no pain will be felt. Because of this knowledge he relaxes and becomes easier to treat. It is for this reason that occasionally a dental surgeon will administer a local analgesic drug for what might well be a painless procedure.

2. Diagnostic purposes

The cause of facial pain is sometimes one of the most difficult conditions to diagnose correctly. This is because the major part of the face receives its sensory supply from the trigeminal nerve which also innervates the jaws, teeth and structures such as the maxillary antra. Severe pain may originate from any of these and it may be impossible for the patient to localize accurately, possibly because of the phenomenon of *referred pain*. When a nerve has several branches, pain originating from a structure innervated by one branch may be misinterpreted by the patient as being localized in another structure innervated by a different branch. Diagnostically, the problem facing the dental surgeon arises because, for example, an abscess in a mandibular premolar may cause symptoms of acute pain in a maxillary tooth on the same side. Fortunately, pain from a lesion innervated by the trigeminal nerve is not referred across the midline so that if the patient complains of pain on the left side of the face then the lesion causing these symptoms is to be found on that side. The only exceptions to this rule occur in the region of the upper and lower incisors where the innervation is derived from a network of nerves from both sides.

Local analgesia can be very helpful with some diagnostic problems because if an injection is given to block nerve conduction in a particular region and the pain is relieved, then it can be deduced that the causative lesion is in the tissue innervated by that nerve.

3. To reduce haemorrhage

Strictly, this is not the use of a local analgesic but of the vasoconstrictor drug which usually accompanies it. However, this use is mentioned here because a local analgesic solution is a very convenient vehicle for administering a vasoconstrictor. It may be of use during surgery under general anaesthesia as it is much simpler to operate in a field where vision is not obscured by blood. The presence of the analgesic in the solution is very desirable, as drugs such as lignocaine tend to prevent cardiac arrhythmia occurring.

Another use of a vasoconstrictor is to control postextraction haemorrhage. An injection of local analgesic solution is given into the soft tissues surrounding the socket and this will eliminate pain from the region and also reduce or stop the haemorrhage by constricting the vessels in the area. This permits the dental surgeon to examine the socket carefully to assess whether further treatment, such as a suture or haemostatic dressing, is required before the effects of the vasoconstrictor have worn off.

4. In conjunction with sedation techniques

Nervous patients may become more confident and relaxed if sedation techniques such as the 'relative analgesia' method of Dr Langa in which nitrous oxide with high concentrations of oxygen is inhaled, or intravenous techniques which are basically a form of intravenous premedication followed by an injection of local analgesia, are used. The sedation technique relaxes the apprehensive patient and the local analgesic ensures that the treatment is painless. With these techniques, which are described in Chapter 13, the patients remain conscious and cooperative with the protective reflexes fully maintained and thus they are not subject to some of the hazards which may be associated with general anaesthesia.

ADVANTAGES OF LOCAL ANALGESIA OVER GENERAL ANAESTHESIA

1. Safety

Local analgesia is safer than general anaesthesia. Although it is uncommon for a fit patient to die because of the administration of a general anaesthetic, it is extremely rare for a fatality to occur from local analgesia, and this aspect is discussed further in Chapter 4.

2. Ease of administration

The administration of a general anaesthetic by a dental surgeon who is also going to carry out treatment on the patient at the same time is a procedure which is to be deprecated. Very special circumstances may occur where this cannot be avoided, but these are few. In the UK a coroner could be highly critical of someone working under these conditions if any mishap occurred to the patient, and thus two qualified persons are required for safe treatment. This opinion was confirmed in June 1975 when the then Chief Dental Officer of the Department of Health, Mr G. D. Gibb, wrote to all National Health Service dentists informing them that the Standing Dental Advisory Committee had advised against operator-administered general dental anaesthetics. The letter stated, 'I accordingly appeal to any in the profession who may still be following the practice to cease it (unless exceptionally it can be justified in extreme emergency) in the interests of their patients and themselves'. This philosophy has now become established practice.

The administration of a local analgesic usually entails the dental surgeon injecting a small quantity of solution into the oral tissues and then waiting for a few minutes until this has achieved the desired result before continuing treatment. Comparing this with the administration of a general anaesthetic, it will be seen that local analgesia is a very much simpler procedure. Under general anaesthesia pain elimination and treatment are performed simultaneously, whereas under local analgesia the procedure of pain elimination is followed by that of treatment.

Normally, local analgesia imposes no restrictions on the patient either before or after its administration, and also has the advantage over general anaesthesia that the patient does not have to fast beforehand. Most anaesthetists recommend that their patients have nothing to eat or drink for at least 4 hours prior to a general anaesthetic. With local analgesia it is advantageous if the patient has eaten beforehand to reduce the likelihood of fainting during treatment.

Local analgesia is less costly than general anaesthesia because it does not involve the payment of a separate fee for the services of an anaesthetist, and there is normally no need for the patient to remain in order to recover after treatment has been completed.

3. Cooperation of the patient

If a patient has a general anaesthetic then it is impossible to obtain the help from him which would normally be available under local analgesia, and there are many occasions during dental treatment when it is very desirable to have that cooperation. An example is the checking of the contour of a newly inserted filling by getting the patient to occlude.

4. Unlimited operating time

Most general anaesthetics administered to outpatients last only for a few minutes and hence the dental surgeon is unable to carry out prolonged operative procedures. With the progress in modern anaesthesia this situation is altering, nevertheless outpatient general anaesthesia still tends to be used mainly for treatment which can be performed quickly.

With local analgesia, the operating time available for the dental surgeon is limited only by the patient's ability to sit still and cooperate. If the effects of the local analgesic are wearing off before treatment has been completed then it is a simple matter for the dental surgeon to inject a further quantity. A patient will usually tolerate conservative treatment for a longer period than oral surgery. Whenever possible, complex surgical treatment should always be done under general anaesthesia with the patient being treated as a hospital inpatient.

5. Reduced bleeding during surgical treatment

As discussed earlier, most local analgesic solutions contain a vasoconstrictor which, besides prolonging the action of the analgesic, also reduces the severity of the haemorrhage which would usually occur during surgical treatment.

6. When the patient is unfit for a general anaesthetic

In these circumstances local analgesia is of particular value. The fitness requirements prior to the administration of a general anaesthetic are far stricter than for local analgesia and they should also be more stringent for an outpatient than for an inpatient. Some of the criteria which lead to general anaesthesia being considered undesirable are:

a. Airway problems, such as nasal obstruction due to deflected nasal septum or nasal polypi, micrognathia, Ludwig's angina, and infections predisposing to oedema of the glottis.

b. Respiratory infections, such as coryza, pneumonia, bronchitis, bronchial asthma, pulmonary tuberculosis and bronchiectasis.

c. Cardiovascular disease which is severe enough to cause dyspnoea at rest, ankle oedema and engorgement of the neck veins.

d. Mechanical problems, such as inability to flex the cervical spine, and conditions in which there is difficulty in opening the mouth, such as trismus or muscle spasm, ankylosis of the temporomandibular joint or obstruction due to neoplasm.

e. Sickle-cell anaemia, which is a severe familial anaemia occurring in Negroes, characterized by sickle-shaped red cells in the blood (*Fig.* 2.1). This affects a patient's fitness for general anaesthesia far more than other anaemias, as even mild hypoxia will stimulate the formation of the abnormal sickle cells and these will obstruct the small vessels and capillaries thus causing serious tissue damage due to infarction. These patients also have very poor wound healing. It should be remembered that if the anaemia is severe then, whatever its type, general anaesthesia will be contraindicated.

Relative indications for avoiding outpatient general anaesthesia are conditions such as pregnancy during the first 3 months and last month

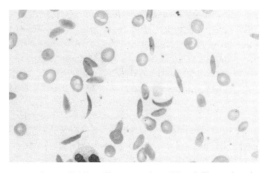

Fig. 2.1. Sickle-cell anaemia. Blood-film showing abnormal-shaped red cells.

to reduce the risks of abortion and premature labour respectively, these risks being dealt with better if the patient is admitted. Some of the other patients who should be admitted are those with a history of coronary thrombosis, and those receiving systemic steroids, who may include the rare group of insulin-resistant diabetics.

FURTHER METHODS OF CONTROLLING DENTAL PAIN

These are lesser used methods which have been employed to achieve pain-free dental treatment in the conscious patient.

1. Acupuncture analgesia

This type of analgesia is thought to have originated in China about 3000 or more years ago and there are records of it being used during the Classical Age (600 BC–AD 200), which is considered to have been a prosperous period in Chinese history.

The term 'acupuncture' is derived from the Latin words *acus,* a needle, and *punctura,* a puncture. The Chinese have used acupuncture as a type of therapy for many medical conditions, and also for analgesia or pain blocking when the acupuncture needles are inserted at various sites on the body based on the ancient meridian theory. Western science now accepts the analgesic aspects of acupuncture but believes that these are largely independent of the precise positioning of the needles at the points determined by ancient Chinese practice. The needles are twirled at 100–120 cycles/min, or instead stimulated by an electrical acupuncture machine which uses a current of about $3\,\mu A$ at a frequency ranging from 300–3000 cycles/min (*Figs.* 2.2–2.5).

Acupuncture analgesia is not always successful but there is no doubt that some patients are able to undergo quite major surgery in comparative comfort using only acupuncture. With this type of analgesia the patient remains completely conscious, and there is no disturbance of the normal physiological functions as there would be during the administration and subsequent recovery period associated with an orthodox general anaesthetic. The mechanism of acupuncture analgesia is not understood well, but one theory has suggested that the needles excite mainly A delta fibres in the peripheral nerves. Inputs from these fibres reach the periaqueductal grey matter and other

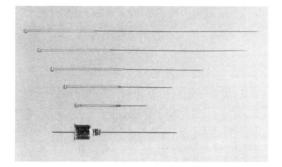

Fig. 2.2. Acupuncture needles shown with a 27-gauge 42 mm long dental hypodermic needle for comparison. The acupuncture needles are not hollow and are very fine.

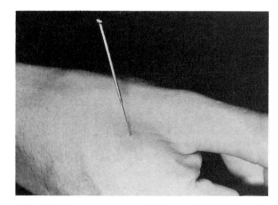

Fig. 2.3. Acupuncture needle inserted in the hand to produce analgesia in the jaw. (*Figs.* 2.3–2.5 are reproduced by courtesy of Dr Neill W. Kerr.)

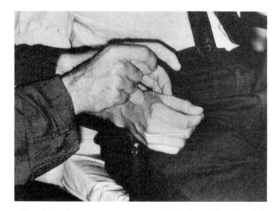

Fig. 2.4. An acupuncture needle being stimulated by twirling it.

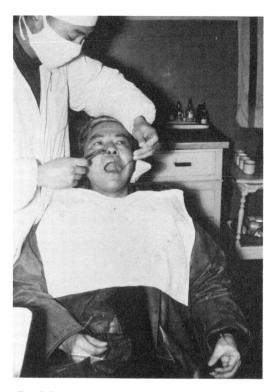

Fig. 2.5. A tooth being extracted under acupuncture analgesia produced by the two needles in the hands.

related structures in the brainstem, thus stimulating the production of endogenous opioids such as endorphins. This view is supported by the reversal of the acupuncture analgesia which usually occurs when the opiate antagonist naloxone is administered (Bowsher, 1980).

2. Hypnotism

Hypnotism is sometimes employed to reduce dental pain in susceptible patients. Initially, the induction of a hypnotic state may be a time-consuming process, but as the patient becomes increasingly conditioned hypnosis will become much more quickly induced. Hypnotism produces a trance-like state in which the patient's attention is focused on the operator so that awareness of other stimuli such as pain is markedly reduced, or not appreciated at all. This makes dental treatment much easier, even when the additional help of a local analgesic injection is required. The use of hypnosis may change a very difficult patient into one who will readily accept treatment.

The disadvantages of this method of pain prevention are that initially it may be time-consuming and also that it does not work for all patients. Other objections are that it is a technique which is not properly understood and some patients may dislike the thought that their behaviour might be controlled or influenced by another person.

3. Audio-analgesia

This is a method of analgesia, described by Gardner and Licklider in 1959, in which the use of loud sounds is said to produce insensitivity to pain in some patients.

A common technique would be one in which the patient wears stereophonic earphones and controls the volume and type of sound—which could be music or a rushing, roaring noise derived from 'white sound' and resembling the sound of sea waves or a waterfall. The patient, having selected a programme of music to induce relaxation, will adjust the volume to a comfortable level and then increase it when the tooth becomes uncomfortable. If the discomfort becomes worse, then the sea noise may be used to eliminate or drown out the pain. Exposure to excessive noise may be dangerous and hence safety standards for audio-analgesia equipment have been recommended by the American Dental Association Council on Dental Therapeutics.

It is possible that audio-analgesia depends to some extent on the suggestibility of the patient. Certainly the music will aid relaxation as it diminishes the noise of the dental drill, and the action of the patient in controlling the choice and volume of sound will divert attention from the actual dental treatment. When both the music and water noise are selected, then the patient will need to concentrate in order to hear the music and this will minimize the awareness of the dental treatment. Physiologically, the pain and auditory pathways are closely associated in the reticular formation and lower thalamus with interactions which are largely inhibitory. The suppression of pain sensation by marked stimulation of another sensory pathway is a common occurrence, possibly due to cross-sensory masking of pain impulses, and this could be an explanation of how audio-analgesia works. However, the appreciation of pain is a complex psychophysiological phenomenon and as yet a simple explanation of audio-analgesia is not possible. The wider use of audio-analgesia has not occurred because it is not effective for all patients and also there may be a problem in communicating with the patient.

4. Electric anaesthesia or anelectrotonus

In 1950, Professor K. Suzuki described a method of blocking nerve conduction in the peripheral part of the pain pathway, by use of a direct electric current. The physiological basis of this type of anaesthesia is that a pain impulse is accompanied by a negative potential and depolarization of the nerve fibre is prevented by introducing a positive potential due to a direct electrical current.

This method of pain prevention has been recommended usually only for the conservative treatment of teeth. A carious tooth has an electrical resistance reported as ranging from $27\,000$ to $2\,300\,000\,\Omega$ and being smallest with incisors and greatest with molars. To achieve anaesthesia with this method, which has no time-lag and produces immediate desensitization, it is necessary to keep the tooth moist, otherwise the electrical conductivity of the system is reduced and anaesthesia ceases.

A paper by A. I. Rybakov and T. V. Nikitina from the Russian Central Research Institute of Stomatology reported on the treatment of 16 500 carious cavities in 7320 patients ranging from 8 to 60 years. It was found that the best results were obtained in children up to the age of 10 years when 92 per cent were successful, and between the ages of 20 and 40 years when 75 per cent were successful, while practically no effect was obtained in patients over 50 years old, these results being assessed by means of pupil and skin-galvanic reactions. These authors recommend the combination of electric anaesthesia with premedication.

A Russian form of the apparatus was the 'Elos-1' machine which was powered by 18-V batteries. It was fixed to the head rest of the dental chair with the anode being connected to the dental handpiece, which had an insulating sheath, and the cathode being clipped on the lobe of the patient's ear. The apparatus did not need to be earthed and the current applied to the tooth was unlikely to exceed 30 mA.

For a time the German firm of Siemens produced a similar apparatus powered by 6-V batteries and having the cathode attached to a saliva ejector instead of the patient's ear, the circuit used being shown in *Fig.* 2.6. The cumbersome Siemens equipment is no longer marketed, as the results obtained from it were unsatisfactory.

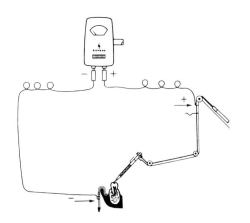

Fig. 2.6. Diagram showing the circuit used by the Siemens apparatus for producing electric anaesthesia.

5. Anaesthesia by cold air

It has long been appreciated that when a part of the body becomes sufficiently cold, pain sensation is abolished due to the inability of nerve fibres to conduct action potentials at low temperatures. Although the dependable reversible cooling of terminal nerve filaments or whole nerves presents considerable practical problems, this principle has been used in the Nondolor apparatus which was produced in France.

It is claimed that the Nondolor apparatus compresses air, cools it, and then dehydrates and sterilizes it with ultraviolet rays. The works are contained within a mobile metal cabinet and the cold air may be applied by means of a pistol with a glass nozzle. The normal rate of delivering compressed air is 60 litres per min which may be at a temperature varying from 35 to 1 °C.

The technique recommended for using the Nondolor is to lower the temperature of the tooth progressively from 35 to 4 °C by projecting the air stream on to the tooth. When this cooling has been achieved, then anaesthesia will begin and the operator should continue to lower the temperature to 1 °C and maintain it at that level. This takes about 3 minutes for incisors and a little longer for posterior teeth. It is essential that the dental treatment is done in absolutely dry conditions and anything such as the tongue, cheek or operator's finger touching the tooth should be avoided, as otherwise cooling will be disturbed. The flow of cold air on the tooth has to be maintained throughout treatment.

This method of anaesthesia has some disadvantages. The tissues become very dry and hence articles such as cotton-wool rolls will stick to the mucous membranes and cause painful ulcers unless the rolls are moistened prior to removal. Also, very sensitive teeth may need a protective covering such as a temporary filling material prior to being cooled, the makers advising that vital teeth with large metallic fillings or crowns may require similar protection. The tooth being treated cannot be cleaned with a water spray or the anaesthetic effect of the cold air is lost, and also the drilling or grinding has to be done in very short stages to avoid generating heat. These disadvantages appear severe enough to discount the use of this method of pain prevention in dental surgeries.

REFERENCES AND FURTHER READING

Bowsher D. (1980) Central mechanisms of orofacial pain. *Br. J. Oral Maxillofac. Surg.* **17**, 185.

Kerr N. W. (1973) The life and work of the dental surgeon and oral surgeon in the People's Republic of China. *Br. J. Oral Surg.* **11**, 36.

Macdonald A. J. R. (1977a) The origins and evolution of medical acupuncture. *Mims Magazine* Issue 46, 83.

Macdonald A. J. R. (1977b) Modern approaches to medical acupuncture. *Mims Magazine* Issue 47, 67.

Man Pang L. (1974) *Handbook of Acupuncture Analgesia* FieldPlace Press, Woodbury, New Jersey.

Weisbrod R. L. (1969) Audio analgesia revisited. *Anaesthesia Prog.* **16**, 8.

Chapter 3

HOW A LOCAL ANALGESIC WORKS

Before discussing the way in which local analgesia prevents a patient feeling pain, it is necessary to consider the nature of pain and the way in which its impulses reach the brain.

Pain is essentially an abnormal affective state that is aroused by the pathological activity of a specific sensory system. It has proved difficult both to define and investigate; however, it is known that it is subserved by its own network of nerve fibres. The cell bodies of these fibres lie in the posterior root ganglia of the spinal cord, or, in the case of the cranial nerves, their respective sensory ganglia. It is to the cells in the spinal nucleus of the fifth cranial nerve that all impulses from the pain receptor nerve endings in all the oral or facial tissues are delivered, irrespective of whether these impulses enter the brain through the trigeminal, the vagus, and possibly the facial and glossopharyngeal nerves. Fibres from the cells in the spinal nucleus of the trigeminal nerve ascend to reach the thalamus, approximately half crossing the midline before they do so. From the thalamus the tertiary

neurons send their fibres to the cerebral cortex (*Fig.* 3.1). The central interpretation of pain is by no means fully understood at the present time, but it may be considered to be an emotional disorder and is always interpreted as coming from a specific area of the sufferer's body, although this may well be incorrect.

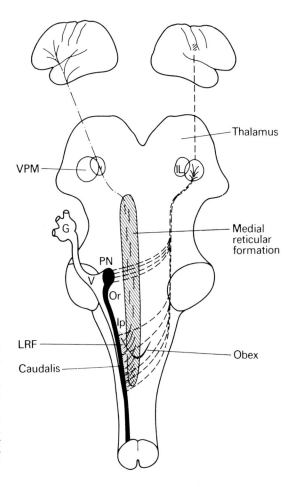

Fig. 3.1. Diagram illustrating the central projections of the pain afferent fibres from the orofacial tissues. G, Gasserian ganglion. V, sensory root of trigeminal nerve. PN, principal sensory trigeminal nucleus. Or, oral subdivision of descending trigeminal nucleus. Ip, interpolar subdivision of descending trigeminal nucleus. Caudalis, caudal subdivision of descending trigeminal nucleus. LRF, lateral reticular formation. VPM, ventroposteromedial thalamic nucleus. IL, intralaminar thalamic nuclei. The broken dotted line represents projections from the principal and descending sensory trigeminal nuclei to VPM, and thence to the orofacial area of the cortex in the postcentral gyrus. The broken line represents projections from the caudal descending trigeminal nucleus via LRF to medial reticular formation, and thence to IL; the latter in their turn give rise to the diffuse thalamocortical projections. (Reproduced by courtesy of Dr D. R. Bowsher and the Editor of the *British Journal of Oral Surgery* (1980) **17**, 187.)

12

PAIN THRESHOLD

This is the level at which pain first becomes perceptible; there is, however, a great variation between different individuals and even the same person at different times. Thus a sportsman may injure himself quite badly during a game but be unaware of this until play is over, whereas normally he would have felt the pain immediately. Conversely, someone who has had no sleep for many nights is liable to be particularly sensitive to the slightest discomfort.

NOCICEPTIVE RECEPTORS

Nociceptive (pain) receptors consist of non-myelinated nerve endings without any specialized structure which may be affected by most stimuli if of sufficient intensity. These nociceptors are widely distributed, being present in the skin, viscera, muscles, dental pulp and periodontal tissues. These receptors possess small nerve fibres which are either myelinated or non-myelinated. The conditions which will give rise to pain occur when the tissues are inflamed, traumatized, necrotic or ischaemic.

The exact manner in which the afferent impulses, which may give rise to pain, are initiated is not fully understood, but depolarization of the receptor endings is caused either directly by chemical or mechanical stimuli or indirectly by what are known as pain-producing substances (PPS). These include K^+ ions, lactate, 5-hydroxytryptamine, bradykinin and histamine. Prostaglandins are released by nerve stimulation and are believed to intensify the effects of the chemical mediators of inflammation such as 5-hydroxytryptamine, bradykinin and histamine.

THE NERVE CELL

The nerve cell or neuron consists of a nucleated cell body and processes. The nucleated body is situated in a site such as the central nervous system (CNS) or a ganglion. Several processes radiate from the neuron, the main one being the axon which is usually very long; the remainder, known as dendrites, are short and are involved in synaptic linkages with axonal terminals. In the peripheral nervous system the axon is covered by layers of supporting cells called Schwann cells which are applied directly to its external surface (*Fig.* 3.2).

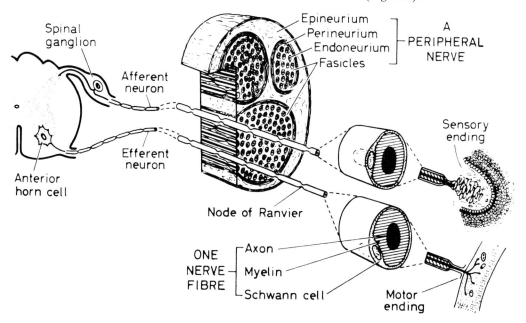

Fig. 3.2. Diagram of the constituents of a mixed peripheral nerve. (Redrawn and modified from Ham A. W. (1957) *Histology,* 3rd ed. London, Pitman.) (From Wyke B. D. (1969) *Principles of General Neurology.* Amsterdam, Elsevier, p. 48.)

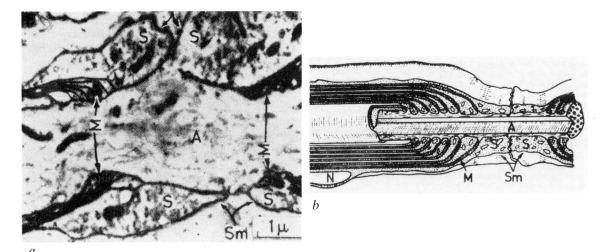

a

b

Fig. 3.3. *a.* Electron photomicrograph of a longitudinal section through a node of Ranvier in a mouse sciatic nerve fibre. The arrows (Sm) indicate the adjoining surface membranes of contiguous Schwann cells. Note that the black-stained myelin lamellae within each Schwann cell (M) stop short on either side of the junction of the Schwann cell membranes, leaving the nodal segment of the axon (A) covered by parts of the Schwann cells (S) devoid of such lamellae. Compare with *b.* Magnificiation indicated by scale. (From Geren Uzman B. and Nogueire-Graf G. (1957) *J. Biophys. Biochem. Cytol.* **3**, 589.) *b.* Diagrammatic interpretation of the electron photomicrograph in *a.* Myelin lamellae (M) are cross-hatched. Stippled areas (S) represent the cut surfaces of the Schwann cell cytoplasm; (Sm) is the Schwann cell membrane; (N) is the Schwann cell nucleus; (A) is the nodal segment of axon. (Redrawn from Geren Uzman B. and Nogueire-Graf G. (1957) *J. Biophys. Biochem. Cytol.* **3**, 589.) (From Wyke B. D. (1969) *Principles of General Neurology.* Amsterdam, Elsevier, p. 17.)

The nerve fibres which are larger than about $2\,\mu$m in diameter are surrounded by a fatty layer of myelin lamellae, the thickness of which increases in direct relation to the size of the axon. Thus, a nerve $10\,\mu$m in diameter would have approximately 80 layers of myelin. The myelin lamellae are laid down by the Schwann cells and are of consistent thickness. Therefore, any increase in the thickness of the myelin layer is brought about by an increase in the number of lamellae. The myelin layer is interrupted at regular intervals, these points being called the 'nodes of Ranvier' (*Fig. 3.3*).

The larger the nerve, then the greater is the distance between consecutive nodes of Ranvier. The actual length of the unmyelinated portion varies inversely with the diameter of the axon, and thus in small myelinated nerves it may be up to $1\cdot5\,\mu$m whereas in the larger diameter ones it is much shorter. The nerve fibres are grouped together in bundles bounded by the fibrous perineurium, and a nerve trunk is formed from several nerve bundles.

MYELIN LAMELLAE

The function of the myelin lamellae is to insulate the nerve fibres and thus, as explained below, to allow more rapid conduction. The presence of the myelin also diminishes the likelihood of a nerve fibre stimulating one of its neighbours with which it may come into contact by acting as a physical insulator. A breakdown of the sheath of motor fibres, as occurs in the demyelinating diseases, causes loss of motor control.

The nodes of Ranvier are points along the nerve fibre at which the myelin is absent, and it is at these sites that ionic exchange normally occurs. Thus conduction in myelinated fibres proceeds in a saltatory or jumping manner from one node to the next and therefore is faster as the action potential does not have to progress slowly down the fibre as a continuously spreading impulse. It is also at these nodes that local analgesics gain access to myelinated nerve fibres and produce their main pharmacological effects.

IMPULSE CONDUCTION

The basic characteristic of nerve cells is their ability to transmit electrical charges, known as nerve impulses, along their entire length. These impulses, once initiated, are self-propagating.

A certain minimal stimulus, termed the 'threshold stimulus', is required to effect a shift in the ionic balance in the nerve fibre and trigger off an impulse, after which there is a refractory period. No further increase in the stimulus will make any difference to the conduction of an impulse in that particular nerve fibre because the size of an impulse transmitted along a nerve cannot vary. However, continuous stimulation leads to a volley of impulses, and an increase in the stimulus may well affect a larger number of fibres and thus augment the number of impulses reaching the brain. Hence the excitability of a nerve increases with its diameter, as the larger diameter nerve will contain more fibres. The largest myelinated peripheral nerve fibres will respond to a weak electrical stimulus, but it is only when the intensity of the stimulus is increased that progressively finer diameter nerves are activated until finally all fibres of the nerve are conducting impulses.

Like all living cells the nerve cell has different concentrations of electrolytes on the inside and the outside. The effect of this concentration gradient of ions across the cell membrane is to produce a potential difference between the inside and the outside of a nerve cell which is normally between 50 and 80 mV, and is known as the 'resting potential'.

Within the nerve cell the concentration of K^+ ions is some 25 times greater than that in the interstitial fluid. However, the intraneuronal concentrations of Na^+, Cl^- and Ca^{++} ions are low, for example, the Na^+ ion concentration being only one fifteenth of that present in the interstitial fluid. There is a continuous ion exchange of K^+, Cl^- and, to a lesser extent, Na^+ ions between the tissue fluid and the neuronal cytoplasm, the ions passing through the surface membrane of the axon via separate ionic channels.

The resting potential of the neuron and its axon depends on maintaining an uneven distribution of electrically charged ions between the interior of the neuron and the tissue fluid surrounding it. With positively charged sodium ions, there is normally a large electrochemical gradient from the exterior to the interior of the neurons. Thus the natural tendency of the sodium ion would be to diffuse inwards more rapidly than out. However, this is balanced by the continuous expulsion of sodium ions from the resting neuron which is achieved by a continuous release of energy within the cell in the form of a Na^+/K^+ pump which also corrects for K^+ leakage. The main source of this is the oxidative metabolism of foodstuffs such as glucose which is taken up from the blood.

When an impulse is conducted the potential at a given point of the nerve fibre changes momentarily from -70 mV to $+20$–30 mV and this change progresses along the nerve. The change in potential is brought about by sodium ion immigration being made possible by a sudden increase in the permeability of the diffusion barrier to these ions which can be initiated by applying a depolarizing current to the neuron. This reversal of the nerve membrane resting potential produces what is known as the 'action potential', and the process is a 'depolarization'.

The outer surface of a resting nerve fibre is positively charged, and the actual conduction of a nerve impulse is due to the stimulated part of the outer nerve membrane becoming briefly electrically negative relative to the unstimulated parts adjacent to the point of stimulus, thus causing a current to flow (*Fig.* 3.4). The opposite occurs on the inside of the cell. Thus to summarize, during impulse conduction an ionic exchange takes place, the Na^+ ions entering the cell and the K^+ ions passing more slowly outside. This produces a very rapid change in potential lasting about 1·5 ms, and it is this depolarization which travels along the nerve

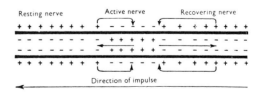

Fig. 3.4. Electrical changes in a nerve fibre during the passage of a nerve impulse. The diagram has been simplified by omitting the Schwann cells. (Reproduced from Anderson D. J. (1952) *Physiology for Dental Students.* London, Edward Arnold.)

and constitutes an impulse, repolarization of the nerve fibre rapidly following.

The manner in which the permeability of a nerve fibre is increased is unknown. However, it is not thought to require the production of any energy by the neurons, this being provided by the external stimulus. It is the repolarization process involving the expulsion of the Na^+ ions which requires energy and this is again provided by the sodium/potassium pump.

If a nerve fibre is stimulated experimentally about half-way along, then the impulse will travel towards both ends. However, a nerve impulse usually travels unidirectionally as the part of the nerve from which the stimulus has just come is recovering from its refractory state. Under normal conditions the impulse produced by stimulation of a motor neuron would not travel far in the CNS, as synaptic transmission is in one direction only, towards the periphery. If a sensory nerve is involved then the synaptic transmission is in the opposite direction, that is towards the brain.

REFERRED PAIN

In certain circumstances pain arising from one region of the body, usually deeply placed and from which impulses are rarely appreciated such as the viscera, is referred either partly or completely to another, usually more superficial, region of the body. This may be due to the relatively poor innervation of the region, but is probably also because the cerebral cortex has not built up an image of the region involved through lack of previous experience. Thus when impulses arising from deeper structures converge on the same spinal neuron as stimuli from a superficial area which is frequently passing impulses, the cortex assumes these impulses are coming from the site from which it is accustomed to receiving stimuli, and hence misinterprets them.

With superficial parts such as the skin, misinterpretation is unlikely to occur as the impulses from nociceptive afferent fibres (those transmitting impulses which are interpreted centrally as pain) are supported by impulses from the mechanoreceptors which assist the brain in interpreting the source of the pain.

In regions such as those innervated by the trigeminal nerve, if impulses received from, say, the mandibular nerve are of sufficient duration and intensity then the cortex becomes unable to determine from which branch the impulses originated. Thus prolonged stimulation of the nerve of a mandibular first molar may produce referred pain which is felt in the maxillary teeth on the same side. However, it is usually possible in these cases to locate the cause of pain by asking the patient where it originated from in the first instance. In the jaws, referred pain never crosses the midline except in the anterior region where there is some slight overlap in the innervation.

SUSCEPTIBILITY TO LOCAL ANALGESIA

To re-establish the resting potential after the passage of an impulse and enable the nerve to continue to function satisfactorily, it needs an adequate concentration of glucose and sufficient oxygen. The nerve also needs certain vitamins, such as thiamine, other substrates such as amino acids and the correct levels of Na^+ and Cl^- ions and other specific substances.

The full details of the mechanism by which the passage of nerve impulses is prevented by local analgesics is unclear, although it is believed that they inactivate Na^+ channels in the nerve fibre membrane and thus prevent inward Na^+ currents from developing. Under these circumstances it is impossible for the membrane to sustain the onward conduction of nerve impulses. Local analgesics raise the threshold for action potentials of the neurons without affecting the resting potential of the neurons or altering their oxygen consumption.

The speed of action and effectiveness of a local analgesic depends on the rate at which it can reach the nerve fibre and build up to a sufficient concentration to attain the critical level at which impulse conduction is prevented. It will gain access to an unmyelinated fibre far more rapidly than one that is myelinated, as the Schwann cells containing myelin are relatively impervious to local analgesics and thus the drug can only act at the nodes of Ranvier where there is no myelin. The smaller the size of a myelinated nerve fibre, the greater the number of nodes per unit length of axon and thus the greater the number of sites at which the local analgesic can act, and therefore the more efficient the analgesia. Similarly, the greater the length of nerve fibre surrounded by the local analgesic, the greater the number of nodes of Ranvier exposed to the action of the analgesic and thus the more rapid the onset of analgesia (*Fig.* 3.5).

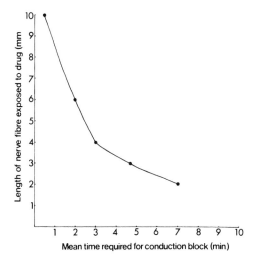

Fig. 3.5. Relation between the time required for the production of conduction block in a single myelinated nerve fibre by a local anaesthetic agent, and the length of nerve fibre exposed to the action of the drug. (Curve constructed from data in Huruyama M. (1941) *Keio Igaku* **21**, 201. Reproduced from Wyke B. D. (1965) in: Evans F. T. and Gray T. C. (ed.), *General Anaesthesia,* 2nd ed., Vol. 1. London, Butterworths, p. 157.)

To reach the nerve, the local analgesic has to migrate from its point of deposition to the site where it will exert its characteristic pharmacological effect. To do this it has to pass through various tissues and interstitial fluid and thus its movement will depend on:

1. The thickness of these barriers such as the epineurium, perineurium and endoneurium (see *Fig.* 3.2).
2. Its solubility in aqueous and lipoid materials.

Very small non-myelinated nerve fibres, such as pain fibres, are affected almost immediately by local analgesics as the drug may act on any site along their length, whereas the only sites of action available in myelinated nerves are at the nodes of Ranvier. In a small myelinated nerve with many nodes per unit length the analgesic still acts fairly quickly, but with large motor nerves with few nodes its action is very slow.

On occasions it will be found that, although soft-tissue analgesia has been obtained, the dental pulp may still be sensitive. This may be because cutaneous afferents are smaller than pulp afferents and thus more susceptible to the local analgesic. The pulp afferents are around 4μm in diameter whereas those supplying the periodontal membrane are around $1 \cdot 5 \mu$m. In the case of the mandibular teeth, additional factors may be (*i*) difficulty of access for the analgesic to reach all the fibres of the inferior dental nerve, particularly when they emerge from auxiliary foramina, usually situated above the mandibular foramen, and (*ii*) that possibly on occasions some innervation is derived from the glossopharyngeal nerve.

Similarly, patients sometimes feel pressure but not pain during extractions because the mechanoreceptive nerve fibres are relatively large and frequently not affected by the local analgesic.

EFFECTIVENESS OF A LOCAL ANALGESIC

The following factors will largely determine the degree of penetration and the effectiveness of the local analgesic.

1. Concentration
The higher the concentration of analgesic, the steeper the concentration gradient and the more rapidly the analgesic will penetrate into the nerve and build up to the level at which impulse transmission is prevented.

2. Solubility
The greater the solubility of the analgesic in both aqueous and lipoid material, the less will be the delaying effect of the tissues and tissue fluids and the more rapid the onset of analgesia.

3. pH of solution
Alkaline conditions favour the anaesthetic crossing the tissue barriers, such as the epi-

neurium, whereas acidic conditions favour the inactivation of sodium channels which produces analgesia.

The higher the pH of the local anaesthetic solution relative to the tissue fluids on the inside of the tissue barrier, the more rapid will be the transfer rate.

Various factors prevent the pH of the solution being raised beyond a certain level. These include:

a. Most analgesics are unstable in alkaline solution.

b. The adverse effect pH would have on the stability of any vasoconstrictor used with the anaesthetic solution.

It is interesting to note that the action of a local analgesic solution is less effective in the presence of inflamed tissues. One suggestion to account for this is that in these cases there is an increased acidity of the tissue fluid which decreases the efficiency of the analgesic, and another possible reason is that the localized vasodilatation accelerates dissipation of the analgesic.

4. Protein binding rate

A rapid protein binding rate produces a quick onset of analgesia, and a rapid separation of the bound protein shortens the time taken for analgesia to wear off and for normal sensation to return. The reverse of these actions occurs with a slow protein binding rate and a slow separation of the bound protein.

DURATION OF ANALGESIA

This depends on the following factors:

1. The amount of local analgesic used. The larger the amount, then the longer it will take for it to be removed by the bloodstream, and for it to be metabolized.

2. The length of time for which the vasoconstrictor usually present in the solution is effective in producing a localized vasoconstriction and thus delaying the removal of the analgesic by the blood. Most local analgesics are smooth-muscle relaxants and thus, when used alone, cause some vasodilatation.

3. An intravascular injection will produce either ineffective analgesia or analgesia of short duration, as a reduced volume of local anaesthetic solution is retained at the intended site of deposition.

4. The rate of metabolism of the local analgesic in the tissues, which may vary with the different types employed, and the speed of its transference from around the nerve fibres to sites such as the liver where metabolism may occur. In some genetic diseases there may be a total lack of breakdown of those local anaesthetics such as the ester type, where metabolic degradation commences in the bloodstream.

Chapter 4
PHARMACOLOGY

Many local analgesic drugs have been discovered but comparatively few of these have found favour in clinical use and the search for the perfect one still continues.

The ideal local analgesic should:

1. Produce complete local analgesia without causing damage to nerve or other tissues.
2. Produce analgesia which is rapid in onset.
3. Produce analgesia of sufficient duration for the treatment planned, but its period of action should not be excessive. For most dental operations 1 hour is adequate.

Although the duration of analgesia depends partly upon the chemical structure of the analgesic, its action is enhanced if it produces vasoconstriction. As this property is usually lacking, it may be compensated for by the addition of a specific vasoconstrictor which reduces the blood flow in the tissues and retards the removal of the analgesic. This is desirable for most operative dentistry, but vasoconstrictors should not be added when obtaining analgesia of structures with a terminal blood supply such as fingers, because ischaemia can occur and result in gangrene.

4. Be non-toxic because it is absorbed into the bloodstream from its site of application.

If two analgesics have the same systemic toxicity but one is more effective at a lower concentration then it will provide the greater margin of safety.

Although an analgesic drug is toxic when its concentration exceeds a certain level in the bloodstream, the addition of a vasoconstrictor such as adrenaline to the analgesic solution permits the administration of a higher safe total dose of analgesic. This is because the vasoconstrictor slows the absorption of the analgesic from the site of application and hence the concentration of analgesic in the circulating blood cannot rise to such a high level. However, if the local analgesic is accidentally injected intravascularly then the presence of a vasoconstrictor will have no effect in reducing the toxicity of the analgesic. An intraosseous injection is made into highly vascular cancellous bone and hence resembles an intravascular injection.

5. Be readily soluble in a suitable vehicle, preferably water.
6. Be stable in solution and have a long shelf-life.
7. Be compatible with the other ingredients in the solution, such as the vasoconstrictor.
8. Be easily sterilized, and this implies that it should not be decomposed by boiling. It is advantageous if the solution is self-sterilizing.
9. Not be habit-forming.
10. Be isotonic and isohydric with the tissue fluids when it is in solution and have a normal pH so that tissue irritation and any subsequent discomfort are minimized.

Local analgesics usually consist of an alkaline analgesic radical combined with a strong acid radical to form a water-soluble salt. For the analgesic action to occur, the salt is hydrolysed on entering the tissues due to the alkalinity of the tissue fluids so that the basic radical is released. This process cannot be aided by making the actual solution alkaline as precipitation of the analgesic would occur and hence the solution would lose its active component. Similarly, it is important that the solution is not too acidic as this inhibits the ionization which liberates the analgesic base. The pH of various analgesics is shown in *Table* 4.1.

In aqueous solutions, local analgesics ionize thus:

$$X = NHCl \rightleftharpoons X = NH^+ + Cl^-$$

(Hydrochloride) salt   Cation Anion

Table 4.1. pH value* of local analgesic solutions

Analgesic solution	pH
Procaine	
Without vasoconstrictor	
2 per cent Novutox† plain	5·5
With vasoconstrictor	
3 per cent Novutox with 1 : 50 000 adrenaline	3·7–3·8
Lignocaine	
Without vasoconstrictor	
2 per cent Xylocaine plain (Astra)	6·05–6·4
2 per cent Xylotox (Pharmaceutical Manufacturing Co. Ltd)	4·2–4·3
2 per cent Lignostab (Boots)	6·1
With vasoconstrictor	
2 per cent Xylocaine with 1 : 80 000 adrenaline (Astra)	3·5–3·55
2 per cent Xylotox with 1 : 80 000 adrenaline (Pharmaceutical Manufacturing Co. Ltd)	4·1
2 per cent Lignostab N with 1 : 80 000 noradrenaline (Boots)	2·6
2 per cent Lignostab A with 1 : 80 000 adrenaline (Boots)	2·0
Prilocaine	
Without vasoconstrictor	
4 per cent Citanest plain (Astra)	5·9–6·3
With vasoconstrictor	
3 per cent Citanest with 1 : 300 000 adrenaline (Astra)	3·6
3 per cent Citanest with 1 : 2 000 000 felypressin (Astra)	4·5–4·7

* Readings obtained using an Electronic Instruments Ltd pH meter.
† Procaine preparation formerly produced by Pharmaceutical Manufacturing Co. Ltd.

and in the tissues which are slightly alkaline, the following reaction occurs:

$$X = NH^+ + Cl^- + NaOH \rightleftharpoons$$
$$\text{(Sodium hydroxide)}$$
$$\text{alkali}$$

$$X = N + NaCl + H_2O$$

where X=N is the alkaline part of the molecule.

The mode of action of the local analgesic is quite complex. It is now considered that the cation is the effective blocker of the axon membrane, thus preventing the passage of sodium ions through the nerve membrane so that nerve impulse propagation is interrupted. However, the alkaline part of the molecule does assist as it is very good at crossing through nerve sheaths. The prevention of the movement of sodium ions stops the excitable nerve membranes from functioning normally and they are said to be 'stabilized' or 'blocked'.

Local analgesics are not so effective in infected tissues. This may be due to the inflammatory vasodilatation flushing the analgesic away from the site of injection, although another possibility is that the presence of pus lowers the pH and thus inhibits the liberation of active analgesic radical.

11. Be free from undesirable side-effects.

The modern local analgesic usually consists of a Ringer's solution to which has been added the local analgesic drug, buffers to maintain the pH, a vasoconstrictor, preservatives, such as the reducing agent sodium bisulphite, which help to prevent the vasoconstrictor from becoming inactivated by oxidation, and an antiseptic such as a paraben, to maintain the sterility of the solution.

The shelf-life of a local anaesthetic cartridge is closely related to the stability of the vasoconstrictor drug which may oxidize and form a dark precipitate. Another source of precipitation occurs when white crystals appear in the solution due to the breakdown of the higher molecular weight portions of the wax which is used as part of the rubber mix in the manufacture of the cartridge plungers. This wax eventually separates from the surface of the rubber and often has a fungus-like appearance although the solution remains sterile.

Local analgesics may produce various pharmacological side-effects following their absorption into the systemic circulation, these varying in degree with the different analgesics.

ACTION OF LOCAL ANALGESICS

1. Action on the cardiovascular system

These actions usually occur only with a relatively high dosage and are primarily a quinidine-like action on the myocardium to give changes in excitability, conduction and force of contraction. Quinidine is a cardiac depressant which reduces the excitability of cardiac muscle, increases the effective refractory period, prolongs the conduction time for the cardiac muscle, and depresses the force of contraction. In addition, most local analgesics produce arteriolar dilatation.

Procaine, procaine amide and lignocaine have all been used intravenously for their quinidine-like effect in controlling cardiac arrhythmias, lignocaine being the present favourite.

Electrocardiographic investigation of outpatients attending Newcastle upon Tyne Dental Hospital suggested that the cardiovascular stress of extractions in otherwise healthy patients, assessed on heart rate and on the occurrence of arrhythmias, is much less under local analgesia than under general anaesthesia. According to the Registrar-General's statistics there were seven occasions on which death occurred following the administration of local analgesia for dental treatment during the period from 1963 to 1976. With some of these the cause of death was related to an underlying medical condition such as a cerebral aneurysm or coronary occlusion.

2. Actions on the central nervous system

All local analgesics stimulate the central nervous system and may produce anxiety, restlessness and tremors. The tremors may even proceed to clonic convulsions which should be treated with sedation by drugs such as barbiturates. If an overdose of local analgesic is administered then death is usually from respiratory failure, partly because there has been excessive central stimulation which has resulted in depression of the respiratory centre, and partly because respiration cannot occur when the intercostal muscles and the diaphragm are in a state of convulsion (*Fig.* 4.1).

The amount of local analgesic reaching the brain depends upon what proportion of the total cardiac output is directed to the brain in the cerebral circulation. For example, if the analgesic is accidentally injected intravenously and at the time of injection the cerebral circulation is the normal 15 per cent of the cardiac output, then the brain accepts 15 per cent of the injected dose. Because the brain is protected by the cerebral blood flow being maintained in adverse circumstances, then there are occasions when the intravascular injection of a local analgesic would be more serious. For example, in a patient with hypovolaemic shock the cerebral blood flow might be as high as 30 per cent of the cardiac output and then the proportion of analgesic reaching the brain would be significantly greater.

Intravenous injections of analgesics are carried via the pulmonary artery to the lungs where much of the analgesic is absorbed by the pulmonary tissue. The concentration of analgesic entering the systemic arteries is much less than that in pulmonary artery blood. The absorption by the lungs may be of short duration, but nevertheless is an important factor in reducing the toxic effects of an intravenous injection. If the local analgesic is injected intra-arterially in the head and neck then the toxic effects are much more serious. The analgesic may enter directly into the cerebral arteries by retrograde flow producing a high concentration of drug in the cerebral circulation, and also the absorption of some of the analgesic by lung tissue does not occur.

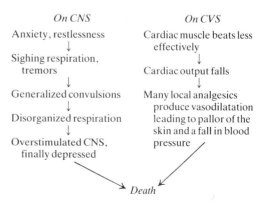

Fig. 4.1. Effects of overdosage of local anaesthesia.

ANALGESIC DRUGS

Cocaine

$$CH_3OOCCH—CH——CH_2$$
$$COO——CH \quad N—CH_3$$
$$CH_2—CH——CH_2$$

This is now only used as a topical surface analgesic but is of historical interest. It is the only analgesic drug commonly used in dentistry which is not synthesized.

Cocaine was the first local analgesic used, largely due to the investigations of Dr Carl Köller in 1884.

It is an alkaloid occurring in coca, the name given to a mixture of dried leaves obtained from plants which are indigenous in Bolivia and Peru (*Fig.* 4.2). When taken orally or sniffed on to the nasal mucosa, cocaine produces exhilaration due to stimulation of the cerebral cortex. It helps overcome fatigue but is very toxic and overdosage results in tremors, convulsions,

hallucinations, myocardial depression and depression of the higher centres. Eventually the medullary centres are affected and death results from respiratory failure which may occur quite suddenly as cocaine is quickly absorbed. The treatment of cocaine poisoning is to inject an intravenous barbiturate to control the convulsions and administer artificial respiration until the respiratory centre recovers.

An extremely important aspect of this drug is that in some people idiosyncrasy may occur, quite a small dosage causing collapse or even death.

Addiction to cocaine leads to emotional, mental and physical deterioration. For these reasons, cocaine must never be used as a local analgesic by injection in dental or oral surgery.

Because cocaine has the serious disadvantage of being habit-forming, it is subject in the UK to the Misuse of Drugs Act, 1971, and Misuse of Drugs Regulations, 1973. A drug in this category is known as a 'Controlled Drug' and this means that a chemist may only supply it to authorized persons or on prescription, its containers are specially labelled, and it is stored in a locked cupboard with a record of its supply noted in a special Controlled Drugs Register.

The regulations regarding prescriptions for this category of drugs are similarly strict. The prescription must:

1. Be in ink or other indelible material.
2. Be dated and signed with the prescriber's usual signature.
3. Be marked 'For Dental Treatment Only' when prescribed by a dental surgeon.
4. Give the prescriber's address, except when provided by a Local Health Authority Service or under the National Health Service.
5. Specify the name and address of the patient.
6. Specify the total amount of the actual controlled drug(s) to be dispensed in both words and figures. There is no provision for 'repeat' prescriptions, but a total amount may be ordered to be dispensed at stated intervals. It is illegal for a dental surgeon or doctor to provide a patient with an incomplete prescription for a Controlled Drug and also the pharmacist is not allowed to dispense it unless the prescription contains all of the requisite information.

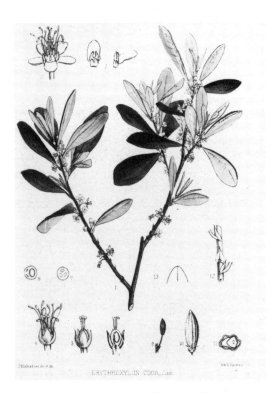

ERYTHROXYLON COCA, *Lam.*

Fig. 4.2. *Erythroxylon coca.* This is the South American plant from which Gaedcke first extracted cocaine. (Reproduced by courtesy of the Wellcome Trustees.)

These statutory requirements emphasize the fact that caution is needed when drugs of addiction are prescribed and that prudent clinical judgement should be used in assessing the correct dosage required for the patient.

Cocaine is effective as a surface analgesic and may be administered in the form of the water-soluble hydrochloride, the dose being up to 8–16 mg or $\frac{1}{8}$–$\frac{1}{4}$ g. It may be used as a 5–10 per cent solution or as a 25 per cent paste, but it is too dangerous for use as an injection because of systemic toxic effects which may even occur due to rapid absorption when used as a surface analgesic. In this form, if the concentration is unduly high, cocaine has been known to produce permanent local damage to the tissues, probably due to ischaemia arising from its action as a vasoconstrictor. This action also delays the absorption of cocaine from the tissues and results in a longer duration of analgesia being achieved than with most of the local analgesics which are vasodilators. The vaso-constrictor-like effect of cocaine is considered to be related to the pyridine ring which is incorporated in its molecule.

Sometimes, when performing an apicectomy on an upper incisor, difficulty may be encountered in obtaining satisfactory analgesia of the tissue forming the apical abscess, granuloma or cyst. For the apicectomy to be successful, it is essential for this pathological tissue to be removed completely. A useful way of achieving analgesia of this region is to soak a cotton-wool roll in 5–10 per cent cocaine solution and then insert this into the patient's nostril on the side on which the apicectomy is to be performed. This is in addition to the routine injections of other local analgesics which would be given into the labial and palatal mucosae adjacent to the tooth.

Research workers modified the structure of the cocaine molecule and discovered other local analgesic drugs. It was frequently found with these synthesized compounds that a particular property such as duration of action, potency or toxicity could be related to modification of a definite part of the cocaine molecule. In this way the research chemists were sometimes able to predict the likely properties of their new products.

Cocaine is the methyl-benzoyl ester of ecgonin and its analgesic properties are due to the ecgonin or to the relationship of the benzoyl and amino groups. Originally, research concentrated on the modification of the benzene ring and although new local analgesics were discovered they still possessed many of the adverse side-effects of cocaine. Because the cocaine molecule breaks down into ecgonin, benzoic acid and methyl alcohol, this led to the investigation of the esters of amino-benzoic acid which achieved more promising results. A further development was the synthesis of procaine, a derivative of *para*-aminobenzoic acid.

Procaine hydrochloride (Novocain, Bayer)

This drug is a very important example of the major group of local analgesics of the ester type which have the general formula:

$$R_1-COO-R_2-N\begin{smallmatrix}R_3\\\\R_4\end{smallmatrix}$$

where R_1 is the aromatic nucleus,

$-COO-R_2-$ is the intermediate chain,

and $-N\begin{smallmatrix}R_3\\\\R_4\end{smallmatrix}$ is the substituted amino group.

It has been found that an increase in the length of the intermediate chain often produces an increase in the analgesic activity. These esters are metabolized by hydrolysis which breaks them down to form alcohols and acids by means of esterases present in the plasma and liver.

Procaine is the diethylamino-ethyl ester of *para*-aminobenzoic acid and its structural formula is:

$$NH_2-\langle\bigcirc\rangle-COO-CH_2-CH_2-N\begin{smallmatrix}C_2H_5\\\\C_2H_5\end{smallmatrix}$$

The hydrochloride, which is water-soluble, has the formula:

$$NH_2-\langle\bigcirc\rangle-COO-CH_2-CH_2-N\begin{smallmatrix}C_2H_5\\\\C_2H_5\end{smallmatrix}\cdot HCl$$

Procaine was synthesized in 1904 by Einhorn and, in the form of the hydrochloride, it has been one of the most widely used local analgesics. For infiltration and block analgesia it is usually employed in the form of a 2 per cent solution. It is of no value as a surface anaesthetic because of its poor rate of absorption from mucous membranes. The discovery of procaine was a great advance on cocaine because although procaine is not as potent, it is very much less toxic.

Procaine is rapidly absorbed from the site of injection, probably because it is a mild vasodilator. In order to prolong the duration of analgesia it is necessary to antagonize this action by using procaine in conjunction with a vasoconstrictor such as adrenaline in a strength of from 1:400000 to 1:50000. In this form the solution of procaine with added vasoconstrictor will produce analgesia within 5 minutes, lasting for between 30 minutes and 2 hours, Procaine is only about one-quarter as toxic as cocaine when administered intravenously or subcutaneously, and for local analgesia up to 400 mg or 20 ml of a 2 per cent solution may be given to a healthy adult. There is an enzyme in the bloodstream and liver, procaine esterase—similar or identical to serum pseudocholinesterase—which aids the hydrolysis of procaine to *para*-aminobenzoic acid, most of which is excreted in the urine.

Procaine is a substance to which susceptible persons may become sensitized. In these people, procaine can cause dermatitis, urticaria and even oedema of the glottis. If a dental surgeon is allergic to this drug then he should avoid employing it. More people have become sensitized to procaine because of the use of procaine penicillin and hence a history of allergy to penicillin may mean that it is dangerous to use procaine. Another side-effect of procaine is that it inhibits the antibacterial activity of the sulphonamides. For this reason, when sulphonamides are prescribed it is unwise to use procaine for inducing local analgesia, for performing lumbar puncture, or for treatment of injuries, otherwise infection may occur. If a patient is on a high dosage of sulphonamides then this tends to prevent the local action of procaine or any of the *para*-aminobenzoic acid derivatives. In this context, it is worth remembering that some of the oral diabetic treatments are based on the sulphonamide molecule and may produce this complication with procaine-type analgesia.

More *para*-aminobenzoic esters

Other local analgesics which are chemically similar to procaine in being esters of *para*-aminobenzoic acid include amethocaine and 2-chloroprocaine.

Amethocaine (Tetracaine, USNF; Anethaine, Glaxo)

$$CH_3-(CH_2)_3-NH\langle\bigcirc\rangle-COO-CH_2-CH_2-N(CH_3)_2$$

The main use of this drug is for producing surface analgesia when a 0·5–2 per cent solution of the hydrochloride is employed. An aerosol spray for dental use is available and each squirt administers about 800 μg. When amethocaine is used as a pharyngeal spray, then up to 8 ml of an 0·5 per cent solution may be used.

If used for dental infiltration or block analgesia then the strength administered is 0·1–0·15 per cent. When used for this purpose it has the disadvantage of diffusing slowly so that the onset of analgesia is delayed. A maximum of 25 mg or 15 ml of a 0·15 per cent solution may be injected for an outpatient.

It is more toxic than procaine but relatively safer as its action is stronger and it may be used in more dilute concentrations. The risk of toxic effects may be further reduced by the addition of a vasoconstrictor, such as adrenaline, to delay absorption.

Sometimes combinations of local analgesics are used for infiltration or block analgesia. One such example is a combination of 2 per cent procaine and 0·15 per cent amethocaine. With this mixture the slow onset of analgesia obtained with amethocaine is compensated for by the more rapid onset due to procaine. Similarly, by the time that the activity of the procaine is on the wane then the amethocaine is producing its maximum effect. There is thought to be no synergistic action with these local analgesic combinations but merely a cumulative effect due to the individual properties of the drugs in the mixture.

2-Chloroprocaine (Nesacaine, Pennwalt, USA)

This is an ester of *para*-aminobenzoic acid but differs from the other local analgesic members of this group already described in having a chloride atom substituted in the benzene ring.

$$NH_2 \text{—} \overset{Cl}{\bigcirc} \text{—} COO\text{—}CH_2\text{—}CH_2\text{—}N \overset{C_2H_5}{\underset{C_2H_5}{}}$$

When structural changes in the chemical molecule are made to produce increased potency of analgesia, then these same alterations usually also increase the toxicity. With 2-chloroprocaine, although the potency is increased to double that of procaine, the rate of hydrolysis is increased to such an extent that it is less toxic than procaine.

2-Chloroprocaine is used as a 2 per cent solution and the total dosage administered should not exceed 800 mg or 40 ml of a 2 per cent solution. Because of its short duration of action due to rapid hydrolysis, it is not used without an added vasoconstrictor. A large-scale trial by Goldman (1969) showed that 2-chloroprocaine was unreliable as a local analgesic and therefore unsuitable for dental use.

meta-aminobenzoic acid esters

Another group of local analgesic drugs is the esters of *meta*-aminobenzoic acid. This group includes *meta*-butethamine and *meta*-butoxy-caine, both of which have been employed for dental use but are seldom used nowadays.

Benzoic acid esters

This group of local analgesics includes pipero-caine, meprylcaine and isobucaine, all of which are esters derived from benzoic acid. Clinically their actions are very similar to those of pro-caine; meprylcaine has a faster onset, and iso-bucaine has a longer duration of action. How-ever, this group of local analgesics is not important as much better drugs are now available.

Benzoic Acid

$$\bigcirc \text{—} COOH$$

Piperocaine (Metycaine, Lilly)

$$\bigcirc \text{—} COO\text{—}CH_2\text{—}CH_2\text{—}N \begin{array}{c} H_2C\text{—}CH_2 \\ | \quad\quad CH_2 \\ HC\text{—}CH_2 \\ | \\ H_3C \end{array}$$

Meprylcaine (USNF) (Oracaine, Oradent)

$$\bigcirc \text{—} COO\text{—}CH_2\text{—}\overset{CH_3}{\underset{CH_3}{\overset{|}{C}}}\text{—}\overset{H}{\underset{C_3H_7}{\overset{|}{N}}}$$

Isobucaine (Kincaine, Oradent)

$$\bigcirc \text{—} COO\text{—}CH_2\text{—}\overset{H_3C}{\underset{H_3C}{\overset{|}{C}}}\text{—}\overset{H}{\overset{|}{N}}\text{—}C_4H_9$$

Anilide non-ester group

This major group of local analgesics is most important as it contains some extremely useful products for dental work. These drugs contain an amide linkage instead of the ester linkage which has been present in the analgesics pre-viously described. They are not affected by the plasma esterases but are mainly metabolized in the liver where the enzymes in the microsomes cause oxidation and de-ethylation, and the end-products are excreted via the kidneys.

It should be remembered that whereas a patient who is allergic to a particular local analgesic drug is likely to be allergic to other analgesics of the same chemical group, it is not so common for the patient to be also allergic to other analgesics in entirely different groups. Hence if a patient has an allergy to 2-chloro-procaine which is an ester of *para*-aminobenzoic acid, then it is worth considering the use of an analgesic of this anilide non-ester group.

The group formula is:

$$R_1\text{—}\overset{H}{\overset{|}{N}}\text{—}\overset{O}{\overset{\|}{C}}\text{—}R_2\text{—}N\overset{R_3}{\underset{R_4}{}}$$

where R_1 is the aromatic residue joined by means of the intermediate chain

$$\text{—NHCO—}R_2 \text{ to the amino group —N} \overset{R_3}{\underset{R_4}{}}$$

The first local analgesic of this type to be used in dentistry was lignocaine, where the aromatic group is xylene.

Lignocaine (Lidocaine, USP; Xylocaine, Astra)

$$\text{CH}_3 \quad \text{H} \quad \text{O} \quad \text{CH}_2-\text{CH}_3$$
$$\text{(ring)}-\text{N}-\overset{\text{O}}{\text{C}}-\text{CH}_2\text{N}\overset{\text{CH}_2-\text{CH}_3}{\underset{\text{CH}_2-\text{CH}_3}{}}$$
$$\text{CH}_3$$

This local analgesic was first synthesized in 1943 by the Swedish chemist Nils Löfgren and then tested by Bengt Lundqvist on himself. Following further evaluation and clinical trials it was released for use in Sweden in 1948 and then later in other countries. This drug has become one of the most widely used local analgesics and is still one of the most effective available.

Experimentally, 10 per cent lignocaine has been injected intramuscularly and has produced similar blood lignocaine levels to those obtained with larger volumes of a 2 per cent preparation. There were no local or general complications associated with the use of a 10 per cent solution in this way and specifically no evidence of any local muscle damage. The strength of solution normally used for local injections in dental work is 2 per cent and up to 10 ml may be administered to an adult, that is a total dosage of 200 mg. If the solution contains a vasoconstrictor then absorption is slower and the maximum total dosage is 25 ml of a 2 per cent solution which is equivalent to 500 mg of lignocaine. These maximum dosage figures are those suggested by the manufacturers, and the higher total quoted when a vasoconstrictor is present assumes that the analgesic solution will remain localized in the tissues and therefore be absorbed more slowly. However, in dental use, accidental intravascular injections sometimes occur and in these cases the vasoconstrictor provides no protection. Because of this risk it is safer to assume that the total dosage for dental work should not exceed 300 mg (15 ml of a 2 per cent solution). Excretion is rapid in the first 3 hours but then the rate of removal falls. Hence the maximum dose should not be repeated too soon, particularly if there is any liver dysfunction, in order to avoid the drug accumulating to a toxic level.

Cannell et al. (1975) reported on circulating levels of lignocaine after perioral injections and their results show that the total dosages of lignocaine used for dental work require careful consideration. The perioral tissues are extremely vascular—a factor which is probably largely responsible for their excellent healing properties. Because of the vascularity of the perioral tissues, injections of lignocaine into them may rapidly produce high levels of circulating drug, and the injection of a maximum of four cartridges (160 mg of lignocaine hydrochloride) frequently produced a circulating level of $1-2\,\mu g$ of lignocaine per ml of plasma. This concentration exceeds the minimum therapeutic level $(1\,\mu g/ml)$ for cardiac treatment stated to be necessary for the control of ventricular arrhythmias. These results suggest that special care should be taken when treating two particular groups of patients who may be affected by prolonged circulating levels of lignocaine within the cardiac therapeutic range. The first group is those patients who have suffered a previous myocardial infarct leading to some degree of heart block or slowing of heart rate, and the second group is those patients who have been prescribed another membrane-stabilizing drug such as phenytoin or propranolol.

Experimentally there have been clinical trials of higher concentrations of lignocaine solutions with 1 : 80 000 adrenaline for dental surgery. Rood (1976) reported on the successful use of 1·0 ml of 5 per cent lignocaine for producing satisfactory analgesia of periodontitic mandibular teeth by means of inferior dental nerve blocks, and Lambrianidis et al. (1980) reported on the use of lignocaine solutions of up to 50 per cent administered with jet injectors when the maximum dosage did not exceed 0·42 ml.

For achieving surface analgesia a 5 per cent ointment may be used and enzymes such as hyaluronidase are sometimes added to aid in the absorption of the ointment by the mucous membrane. Lignocaine solution in a concentration of 0·5 per cent may also be used as a mouthwash for achieving surface analgesia.

Lignocaine is an extremely effective drug. It is stable and is able to withstand boiling and also autoclaving. Its analgesic action is very rapid in onset, twice as effective as that achieved by procaine, and also present for a much longer duration; indeed some consider that this is excessive as it may last for about 3 hours. Weight for weight, lignocaine is more toxic than procaine but, as its analgesic action is so much stronger, less is required. As lignocaine has no vasoconstrictive action on terminal arterioles, the addition of a vasoconstrictor is almost essential to reduce its rate of absorption, prolong its action and hence reduce its toxicity. After absorption from the tissues, most of the lignocaine is detoxicated in the liver by amidases and the remainder is excreted unchanged in the urine. It is virtually free from side-effects and is one of the safest local analgesics, although toxic reactions such as nausea, vomiting, muscular twitching and transient drowsiness may occur from accidental intravenous injection. Allergy is very rare. Astra Pharmaceuticals investigated many incidents of alleged allergy to lignocaine and found that in all those cases the allergen was not lignocaine but the preservative in the solution. The preservative belongs to a group of chemicals known as parabens which are widely used in diverse concoctions varying from sauces to cosmetics. Now the Astra company markets paraben-free solutions of lignocaine, and since then they have received markedly fewer reports of side-effects.

Mepivacaine (USP) (Carbocaine, Pharmaceutical Manufacturing Co.)

Mepivacaine is a local analgesic similar to lignocaine and may be used in a 3 per cent solution on its own, or as a 2 per cent solution with 1 : 80 000 adrenaline. The 3 per cent solution has a shorter time of action when used for an infiltration, but there is no evidence of any difference for regional analgesia. Both solutions of mepivacaine produce a shorter duration of soft-tissue analgesia following infiltration than 2 per cent lignocaine with 1 : 80 000 adrenaline, and, after regional analgesia, 3 per cent mepivacaine produces shorter duration of soft-tissue analgesia than either of the other two solutions. Its depth and rate of onset of analgesia are very similar to those of lignocaine, deep analgesia being achieved very rapidly.

Mepivacaine, with or without adrenaline, is a good local analgesic drug. It may have a slight vasoconstrictor action and this could be related to the pyridine ring which is incorporated in its molecule and which is also found in cocaine, another analgesic with vasoconstrictor properties. Mepivacaine without a vasoconstrictor has a 5-year shelf-life, irrespective of the conditions of storage, and this is in contradistinction to local analgesics containing a vasoconstrictor, which should be stored in a cool place to ensure efficiency.

The total dosage of mepivacaine should not exceed 300 mg or 15 ml of a 2 per cent solution. Mepivacaine may be slightly less toxic than lignocaine.

Pyrrocaine (USNF) (Dynacaine, Graham Chemical Corp.)

Pyrrocaine is a local analgesic of the amide type and, like lignocaine and mepivacaine, is an acyl derivative of xylidine. The local anaesthetic properties of pyrrocaine are very similar to those of lignocaine except that it has been reported as having less vasodilating action than lignocaine. It has been marketed as a 2 per cent solution with adrenaline in concentrations varying from 1 : 250 000 to 1 : 100 000 and clinical trials have been made using pyrrocaine with vasopressin as the vasoconstrictor.

Bupivacaine (Marcain, Duncan, Flockhart)

This local analgesic was developed from mepivacaine and is thus related chemically to lignocaine. Bupivacaine differs from mepivacaine in that a methyl group in the piperidine ring has been replaced by a butyl group.

The rate of onset of analgesia with bupivacaine is slower than that of lignocaine and mepivacaine, but it differs from these drugs in producing a much longer duration of analgesia. This is about twice that of lignocaine and hence, if major oral surgery under local analgesia is contemplated, bupivacaine would seem to be the drug of choice. It appears to be a relatively safe analgesic and its use has been reported on patients with cardiovascular disease with no evidence of any harmful side-effects. However, there have been reports of cardiac arrest or ventricular tachycardia, some fatal, particularly associated with extradural blocks administered for pain relief to pregnant mothers during delivery. Severe cardiac complications have also been reported with intravenous injections of bupivacaine. Experiments have demonstrated that cardiovascular collapse occurs at a lower plasma concentration of bupivacaine in the pregnant animal compared with the non-pregnant, and also that compared with lignocaine and mepivacaine, bupivacaine causes more maternal cardiac problems and fetal hypoxia. The variation in cardiotoxicity between different local analgesics may depend upon their ability to block the passage of sodium ions and the duration of this blockage. It is possible that bupivacaine also blocks calcium channels. In view of these reports, it would seem prudent to avoid the use of bupivacaine on pregnant patients and the use of aspirating syringes to avoid the risk of intravascular injections is essential. It is also most important with bupivacaine not to exceed the recommended dosage.

As bupivacaine is approximately four times as potent as lignocaine, it is used as a 0·5 per cent solution which is equivalent to 2 per cent lignocaine. The bupivacaine solution at present available for clinical use has 1 : 200 000 adrenaline added and this increases both the speed of onset and the duration of analgesia. The maximum recommended dosage for a healthy adult in any 4-hour period is 125 mg or 25 ml of a 0·5 per cent solution, although American references have quoted total dosages varying between 90 mg and 175 mg. The slow rate of onset can be compensated for by giving an injection of lignocaine first, although one American trial found no significant difference in onset time when comparing bupivacaine and lignocaine in a double-blind clinical trial.

Prilocaine (Citanest, Astra)

$$\text{NH}-\text{CO}-\underset{\underset{\text{CH}_3}{|}}{\text{CH}}-\text{NH}-\text{CH}_2-\text{CH}_2-\text{CH}_3$$

The most recent of the anilide non-ester local analgesics is prilocaine in which a toluene group replaces the xylene group which is present in lignocaine.

This was first reported in 1960 when it was known as L.67. In experiments on laboratory animals prilocaine was found to be as effective as lignocaine but only 60 per cent as toxic. It has less tendency to accumulate in the tissues, this is due to an increased rate of metabolism as it is broken down directly by hepatic amidase. It seems to have a weaker action on the central nervous system and also differs from lignocaine in possibly being a mild vasoconstrictor.

The results of a clinical trial reported by Goldman in 1965 show that 3 per cent prilocaine with 1 : 300 000 adrenaline has the same effectiveness as 2 per cent lignocaine with 1 : 80 000 adrenaline. With people in good health, the only significant disadvantage of adrenaline or other vasoconstrictors is when accidental intravenous injection occurs. This mishap can be prevented by using an aspirating syringe and checking that a vein had not been entered prior to injecting any solution. Experiments with rabbits have shown that the rise in blood pressure produced by intravenous injection of 3 per cent prilocaine solution with 1 : 300 000 adrenaline is less than half that produced by 2 per cent lignocaine with 1 : 80 000 adrenaline. These findings are presumably related to the much smaller amount of adrenaline in the 3 per cent prilocaine solution and therefore indicate that this might be of value when treating patients with hypertension.

With infiltration injections 3 per cent prilocaine with 1 : 300 000 adrenaline gives analgesia of the soft tissues for a shorter duration than 2 per cent lignocaine with 1 : 80 000 adrenaline. Hence this factor must be considered when choosing which analgesic drug should be used for a particular operation. The speeds of onset were similar for prilocaine and lignocaine, and it has been reported that the incidence of initial pain immediately upon injection was less with the former because of the lower concentration of adrenaline.

Prilocaine causes cyanosis due to methaemoglobinaemia in patients receiving very high dosages. This can be prevented by adding the oxidizing agent methylene blue to the injected solution or by the administration of tablets of methylene blue, 3 g, beforehand. A case of a 5-year-old boy who had an idiosyncratic reaction to prilocaine producing acute toxic methaemoglobinaemia associated with hypoxia and general motor seizures after receiving only 1·3 ml of prilocaine hydrochloride injected intraorally was reported by Ludwig (1981). Quoting from this paper, patients with methaemoglobinaemia levels of 10–20 per cent are cyanotic but tolerate the condition well. At levels of 35–40 per cent patients often experience exertional dyspnoea, headaches, tachycardia and dizziness. Stupor appears around the 60 per cent level, and the 70 per cent methaemoglobinaemia level is probably lethal. Treatment of the acute condition is slow intravenous injection of methylene blue at a dosage of 1–2 mg/kg body weight over approximately 5 minutes, with the dose repeated 1 hour later if cyanosis is still present.

If it is desired to use a local analgesic without a vasoconstrictor then 4 per cent prilocaine may be employed. With infiltration techniques this produces a rapid onset of pulpal analgesia lasting for approximately 15 minutes, and with inferior dental injections, pulpal analgesia is of about 1½ hours' duration, the analgesia again being of rapid onset.

A more recent product is the combination of 3 per cent prilocaine with the vasoconstrictor felypressin, which is several hundred times less toxic than adrenaline. Patients who have an idiosyncrasy or are hypersensitive to synthetic adrenaline and those on antihypertensive drugs can be given felypressin without risk, although in cases of ischaemic heart disease not more than 8·8 ml of this local analgesic solution should be used at one visit. During general anaesthesia using halothane or cyclopropane, felypressin may be safely employed, whereas catecholamines such as adrenaline are contraindicated because of the danger of cardiac arrhythmia.

The manufacturers recommend that the total injected dose should not exceed 600 mg or 20 ml of a 3 per cent solution when combined with adrenaline or felypressin and 400 mg or 13 ml of a 3 per cent solution with a vasoconstrictor. For dental use the total dosage should not exceed 400 mg (10 ml of a 4 per cent solution or 13 ml of a 3 per cent solution) because of the risk of accidental intravascular injections. At these dosages the complication of methaemoglobinaemia should not occur.

Kaliciak and Chan (1986) reported a fatality in Canada when an 83-year-old man was given 12 cartridges containing 864 mg of plain prilocaine over a period of 1 hour for the extraction of 16 teeth. The patient died in the dental surgery in spite of attempts at resuscitation. It was concluded that death was due to prilocaine overdose. The drug concentrations in the tissues were measured about 1½ hours after the initial injection, the values being in the blood 13·4 mg/l, urine 69·4 mg/l and in the liver 49·2 mg/kg. The interpretation of these results was that the blood level confirmed the high dosage injected and the urine level showed good renal evacuation. The report mentioned that rat experiments had demonstrated that following intramuscular injections of prilocaine, the concentration in the organs decreased in the following order: lung, kidney, spleen, brain, heart, liver and blood.

Because of the risks to the pregnant patient and fetus discussed on p. 34, in the section on felypressin, it is wise to avoid the use of prilocaine on pregnant patients.

Butanilicaine Phosphate (Hostacain, Hoechst)

$$\text{Cl} \quad \text{H} \quad \text{O}$$
$$\langle \text{ring} \rangle - \text{N} - \overset{\text{O}}{\underset{}{\text{C}}} - CH_2 - NH - (CH_2)_3 - CH_3 - H_3PO_4$$
$$\text{CH}_3$$

Butanilicaine is another of the anilide non-ester group of local analgesics. It is not such a marked vasodilator as procaine and has a potency almost equal to that of lignocaine.

It has been used in dentistry as a 2 per cent solution mixed with 1 per cent procaine under the tradename Hostacain. Hostacain SP has 1 : 50 000 adrenaline as its vasoconstrictor, whereas Hostacain NOR had 1 : 25 000 noradrenaline. Butanilicaine is rapidly metabolized in the liver by being broken down by peptidase and is eliminated about four to five times as quickly as lignocaine, thus enabling the maximum recommended adult dose to be as high as 1 g. When Hostacain is used on an outpatient not more than 20 ml should be injected. The onset of analgesia is between 2 and 4 minutes and the duration of analgesia is about 40 minutes, Hostacain SP providing a longer duration than Hostacain NOR.

HYALURONIDASE (Hyalase, Fisons)

Hyaluronidase is not an analgesic but an enzyme which is sometimes added to analgesic pastes and solutions. It occurs naturally in the heads of spermatozoa for softening the pellicle of the ovum, and also forms the 'spreading factor' of organisms such as the haemolytic streptococcus and gas-gangrene bacillus. It acts by hydrolysing the viscous polysaccharide complex which binds connective tissue cells together and thus increases their permeability. This hydrolysis is soon reversed so that the intracellular cement substance reforms.

Hyaluronidase is manufactured from bulls' testes and marketed as a powder in ampoules containing 1500 international units (formerly Benger's units); it may be added to local analgesic solutions and pastes to facilitate their diffusion. It is unnecessary to add this enzyme to analgesic solutions used for dental injections.

VASOCONSTRICTORS

The addition of a vasoconstrictor to an analgesic solution temporarily diminishes the local circulation in the tissues and therefore delays the removal of the analgesic. This increases the efficiency and duration of the analgesia (*Fig.* 4.3). Another advantage of the vasoconstrictor is that it reduces the risk of generalized poisoning by the analgesic solution by slowing its absorption into the bloodstream so that it may be more readily detoxicated by the appropriate enzyme.

The local analgesic drug may have an action on the blood vessels. For example, it is claimed that prilocaine with only 1 : 300 000 adrenaline will produce almost as great a vasoconstriction as lignocaine with 1 : 80 000 adrenaline. From the dental viewpoint it may be considered that, of the local analgesics which have been described, cocaine is the only powerful vasoconstrictor, mepivacaine and prilocaine are mild vasoconstrictors, and all the others produce varying degrees of vasodilatation.

Adrenaline (Epinephrine, USP)

$$HO-\underset{HO}{\underbrace{\bigcirc}}-CHOH-CH_2-NH-CH_3$$

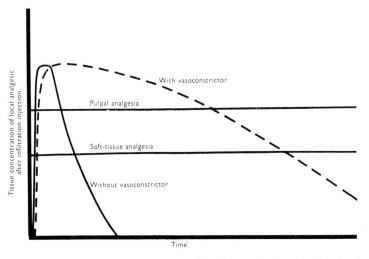

Fig. 4.3. Effect of the addition of a vasoconstrictor drug on the duration of analgesia.

Adrenaline is an active principle of the adrenal medulla and may be either obtained from an extract of mammalian adrenal glands or prepared synthetically. It is stable in acid solution and is used in a concentration varying from 1 : 50 000 to 1 : 300 000 when added to a solution of local analgesic. Both light and 'rubber plasticizers' oxidize adrenaline and therefore it should be kept in dark bottles or ampoules. Multidose bottles with rubber caps cause rapid deterioration of both adrenaline and noradrenaline. In dental cartridges, oxidation of the vasoconstrictor occurs where the solution is in contact with the rubber plunger and a loss of 50 per cent of the vasoconstrictor activity may occur within 18 months to 2 years. The nominal shelf-life of a local anaesthetic cartridge is 2 years, although this may be decreased as a result of storage at high temperatures.

The total dosage for dental use should not exceed 0·2 mg. From a study of 12 fatal cases of adrenaline poisoning, the minimum lethal subcutaneous dose causing death in an adult was 4 mg and the maximum dose tolerated was between 7 and 8 mg. When considering total drug dosages for dental patients, it should be borne in mind that these patients are usually ambulatory and desire to leave the dental surgery immediately after their treatment. Another aspect of vasoconstrictors is that it is very frequently the dosage of these drugs, and not the local analgesic, which imposes the limit upon the total volume of analgesic solution which may be safely administered on one occasion.

The pharmacological actions of adrenaline resemble the responses produced by the stimulation of adrenergic nerves. Some of the effector cells of the sympathetic nerves of the autonomic nervous system are stimulated by adrenaline, while others are inhibited. To simplify our understanding of this, it is assumed that there are two types of receptors at the site of these effector cells. They are known as alpha-receptors if concerned with excitatory effects and beta-receptors if concerned with inhibitory effects. Examples of excitatory actions are vasoconstriction and dilatation of the pupil. Examples of inhibitory actions are vasodilatation of the blood vessels of voluntary muscles and relaxation of bronchial muscles. Adrenaline stimulates both alpha- and beta-receptors and thus it dilates blood vessels in skeletal muscle and myocardium, and constricts those in the skin.

A clinical trial reported by Cardwell and Cawson to the British Division of the IADR in 1969 showed that when used in dentistry with both infiltration and regional nerve block injections, there were approximately half as many failures with a lignocaine solution containing 1 : 80 000 adrenaline compared with a solution containing 1 : 250 000 adrenaline. Galley (1969) considered that for regions outside the vascular area of the mouth 1 : 80 000 adrenaline was probably far too strong and may cause prolonged ischaemia, whereas 1 : 250 000 was effective but harmless.

When operating under general anaesthesia, the surgeon may infiltrate the tissues with a local analgesic solution containing adrenaline to reduce bleeding. The use of a solution containing adrenaline or noradrenaline in these circumstances should not be carried out without the permission of the anaesthetist. This is because some general anaesthetic drugs, such as chloroform, cyclopropane, ethyl chloride and halothane, sensitize the myocardium of the heart to adrenaline so that a marked fall in systolic blood pressure and ventricular fibrillation may result. If the anaesthetist advises against the use of adrenaline in these circumstances then it may be possible to obtain the desired result by using another vasoconstrictor such as felypressin.

If a vasoconstrictor is required to reduce bleeding when operating under general anaesthesia, it is better to use a solution containing a local analgesic of the amine group such as lignocaine than to use the vasoconstrictor drug on its own. This is because the risk of cardiac arrhythmia occuring is thereby greatly reduced, and this is borne out by the fact that in ventricular fibrillation, tachycardia or extrasystoles the treatment is an intravenous injection of a drug such as lignocaine.

Noradrenaline (Levarterenol, USP: Levophed, Winthrop Laboratories)

$$HO \underset{HO}{\overset{}{\bigcirc}} CHOH{-}CH_2{-}NH_2$$

Noradrenaline is a neurohormone present in the adrenal medulla and is also released on stimulation of the postganglionic adrenergic nerve fibres. The pharmacological actions of noradrenaline are almost entirely alpha-receptor effects, that is they have an excitatory action on the effector cells of the sympathetic nervous system. It constricts the blood vessels in skeletal muscle and its action on the heart differs from that of adrenaline.

Noradrenaline is a less effective vasoconstrictor than adrenaline, although the vasoconstriction obtained from noradrenaline lasts longer. Noradrenaline is available in local analgesic solutions in concentrations varying from 1 : 80 000 up to 1 : 25 000 and it has been quoted that for dental use, the total dosage should not exceed 0·34 mg. However, in view of the adverse reactions, including one death, which have been reported in patients who have received injections of noradrenaline 1 : 25 000 concentration, the use of local anaesthetic solutions containing noradrenaline is unjustifiable. Although some of the patients in whom these ill-effects occurred were known to be taking tricyclic antidepressant drugs, it was uncertain whether all of them were. Whereas the predominant action of noradrenaline causes a rise in blood pressure, that of adrenaline results in an increase in the heart rate which is the safer side-effect.

Effects of adrenaline and noradrenaline on the heart

Adverse reactions to these vasoconstrictors are most likely to occur if the drug is accidentally injected intravascularly and therefore an aspirating syringe should be used to minimize the risk of this occurring. The patients most at risk would be those with cardiac disorders, diabetes or thyrotoxicosis, or on drug therapy involving tricyclic antidepressants or adrenergic neurone blocking agents. Aellig et al. (1970) reported transient increases in heart rate of up to 40 beats per minute when injecting 2 per cent lignocaine with 1 : 80 000 adrenaline, but this was when using non-aspirating syringes. This increase of heart rate would probably not matter in a healthy patient but could be hazardous in a patient with cardiac disease.

The effects of these hormones on the cardiovascular system are very complex. Adrenaline by its direct action increases the heart rate and also the force of contraction of the myocardium. These actions together arouse the patient's awareness of his heart beat so that he may complain of palpitations. The cardiac output is increased and this causes a rise in systolic blood pressure. The blood vessels of the skeletal muscles (and those of the heart) dilate and this dilatation causes a decrease in peripheral resistance and thus a fall in diastolic blood pressure.

Noradrenaline causes a rise in systolic and diastolic blood pressure and due to this a reflex slowing of the heart rate occurs. There are minimal effects upon the force of myocardial contraction and cardiac output. The vessels in the skeletal muscles are constricted and it is thought that there is enhancement of the coronary blood flow, but whether this is due to coronary vasodilatation or merely secondary to the other cardiovascular changes is not at present understood. The total peripheral resistance is increased.

To summarize, the amounts of catecholamine vasoconstrictors used in local analgesia are very small and because of their enhancement of the action of the local analgesic then very little solution is required, assuming that the dental surgeon is accurate with his injections. If the dental surgeon is concerned about his patient's cardiovascular system then he may wish to use a local analgesic solution without a vasoconstrictor, but he must remember that much more of the solution will then be required and accurate injections are essential. The duration of effective analgesia varies with the analgesic used, but is appreciably shorter, especially so with infiltration analgesia. It should be remembered that if analgesia is inadequate, far more distress is likely to occur to the patient than would have arisen from the use of a small quantity of local analgesic solution containing a vasoconstrictor.

Nordefrin hydrochloride (Cobefrin)

$$HO-\langle \rangle-CHOH-\underset{\underset{NH_2}{|}}{CH}-CH_3 . HCl$$

(HO, HO on ring)

Nordefrin hydrochloride is a sympathomimetic amine like adrenaline and noradrenaline, and similarly its chemical structure is that of a catechol derivative with two hydroxyl groups in the *ortho* position. Neary all the vasoconstrictive activity is possessed by the laevo isomer, levo-nordefrin (USNF) (Neo-cobefrin).

The vasoconstrictive action of nordefrin hydrochloride is very much less than that of adrenaline and thus when added to a local analgesic solution it is used in the relatively high concentration of 1 : 10 000. The total dosage administered should not exceed 1 mg or 10 ml of a 1 : 10 000 solution. Weight for weight, it is less toxic than adrenaline, but in clinical use, because of the higher concentration necessary, its actual toxicity is similar. There have been several deaths reported from its use on thyrotoxic patients and therefore it should be avoided. Because it is weaker as a vasoconstrictor, it has no material advantages over the more commonly used drugs except that it is more stable than adrenaline or noradrenaline.

Phenylephrine (Neophryn, Neosynephrine, Winthrop Laboratories)

$$HO{-}\langle\ \rangle{-}CHOH{-}CH_2{-}NH{-}CH_3$$

The chemical structure of this vasoconstrictor is similar to that of adrenaline except that there is only one hydroxyl group substituted in the benzene ring.

This drug has sympathomimetic actions similar to adrenaline and noradrenaline. It differs from these drugs in that it is very stable and therefore its duration of pharmacological activity is greater. Its pressor activity is less, although it may be used to treat collapse due to a fall in blood pressure by injecting 2–5 mg intramuscularly or 0·2–0·5 mg intravenously. It lacks the cardiac and adverse central effects of adrenaline and is extremely safe, its relative toxicity being similar to that of adrenaline. It is one of the very few vasoconstrictors which do not cause cardiac arrhythmias, although it may cause a reflex bradycardia. It is thought to dilate the coronary arteries and stimulate the myocardium so that the cardiac output is increased.

In local analgesic solutions, phenylephrine is used in a concentration of 1 : 2500. The total dosage administered for dental purposes should not exceed 4 mg or 10 ml of a 1 : 2500 solution in a healthy adult, and should be much less if the patient has cardiovascular disease.

VASOPRESSINS

There have been many attempts at discovering safer vasoconstrictors than the sympathomimetic amines, adrenaline and noradrenaline. One avenue of research has been to investigate the hormones of the posterior lobe of the pituitary gland, the so-called vasopressins, which include vasopressin, felypressin and ornipressin.

Vasopressin BP (Pitressin, Parke, Davis)

Vasopressin is a naturally occurring substance containing the pressor principle of the posterior lobe of the pituitary gland, and has been used as a vasoconstrictor with the local anaesthetic pyrrocaine which is no longer used. Vasopressin is prepared in the form of a sterile aqueous solution in a fractionation processing of the pituitary glands of oxen or other mammals. The vasopressor activity is measured by an assay method based on the increased arterial blood pressure responses induced in rats which have had their adrenergic responses blocked by drugs. The extract contains not only pressor principle, but also antidiuretic hormone which is used for treating the polyurea which occurs in diabetes insipidus.

The synthetic pressins include felypressin and ornipressin.

Felypressin (phelypressine; PLV2; Octapressin, Sandoz)

Felypressin is a synthetic posterior-lobe pituitary hormone. It is a polypeptide resembling the naturally occurring posterior pituitary hormone, vasopressin, but differs in structure in having phenylalanine substituted in the molecule in place of tyrosine.

The pressor effect of felypressin is smaller than that of adrenaline and of slower onset but may be of longer duration. Its action as a vasoconstrictor is also less than that of adrenaline and there is no accompanying tissue hypoxia as may occur with adrenaline and noradrenaline.

Local analgesics containing felypressin may be safely used in conjunction with general anaesthetics possessing halogenated hydrocarbons and also with cyclopropane without any risk of causing ventricular fibrillation. This contrasts with the increased myocardial sensitivity which occurs when adrenaline or noradrenaline is used in conjunction with cyclopropane and also to a lesser extent with halothane. Felypressin has the great advantage that it may also be safely used for the thyrotoxic patient and for the patient receiving monoamine oxidase inhibitors, although with this latter type of patient many authorities consider that the minute amounts of adrenaline and noradrenaline used in local analgesic solutions present no danger.

Felypressin should not be used for a pregnant patient as it has a mild oxytocic effect which may impede the placental circulation by interfering with the tone of the uterus. This contraindication is made particularly valid by the fact that felypressin is normally available with prilocaine, which also passes the placental barrier, and a high dose might cause fetal methaemoglobinaemia.

There is no problem with giving felypressin to patients on tricyclic drugs. In experiments on anaesthetized dogs, Goldman et al. (1970) showed that there was no potentiation of the pressor action of felypressin in animals which had been pretreated with the tricyclic antidepressant, desmethylimipramine, whereas both noradrenaline and adrenaline caused potentiation.

A combination of felypressin with prilocaine gives a better analgesic effect than a combination with lignocaine. Experimental work in Malmö, Sweden, showed that the optimal combination was 3 per cent prilocaine with 0·03 iu per ml felypressin, a strength equivalent to a 1 : 2 000 000 concentration, and that, contrary to expectation, higher concentrations of felypressin gave less vasoconstriction and a correspondingly shorter duration of analgesia. This unusual finding regarding the concentration of felypressin was not explained (Berling, 1966).

Felypressin has a very low toxicity with an unusually high safety margin. In animal experiments no evidence of coronary ischaemia was found and other experiments to study local tissue irritation showed no differences between solutions containing felypressin and those with adrenaline. It seems extremely likely that felypressin may become the vasoconstrictor of choice if the dental surgeon has any cause for concern regarding the patient's cardiovascular system. The Dunlop Committee on Safety of Drugs (now known as the Committee on Safety of Medicines) has placed no restriction on the use of felypressin for healthy patients but has advised that not more than 8·8 ml of a 1 : 2 000 000 solution should be used in patients known to have ischaemic heart disease, presumably because in high dosage it may cause coronary vasoconstriction leading to tachycardia. This amount is equivalent to the contents of four dental cartridges and exceeds the average volume of local analgesic solution used during a dental appointment. Healthy adult patients should not be injected with more than 13 ml of a 1 : 2 000 000 solution at one visit.

Ornipressin (POR-8, Sandoz)

This is another synthetic posterior-lobe pituitary hormone of the vasopressin type which has been under consideration for dental use. It has been reported that its vasoconstrictor action is comparable to that of adrenaline but it does not have such undesirable side-effects on the blood pressure, heart rate and cardiac rhythm as result from adrenaline and noradrenaline, and it is less toxic than felypressin. There is no contraindication to the use of POR-8 on patients taking tricyclic antidepressants and no interaction between POR-8 and general anaesthetics such as halothane.

POR-8 has been used as a vasoconstrictor with 2 per cent mepivacaine, the vasoconstrictor being in concentrations of 0·03 iu/ml and 0·05 iu/ml. Both of these concentrations were found to be satisfactory, although 0·03 iu/ml was considered to be the lowest acceptable strength. There was no suggestion that the analgesic effect varied inversely with the vasoconstrictor concentration, as had been reported with felypressin–prilocaine mixtures. The POR-8 acted approximately as rapidly as adrenaline and more quickly than felypressin, but the greatest vasoconstrictor effect of the POR-8 did not occur until about 10–15 minutes after its administration. The total dosage should not exceed 2 iu, and it would be most unlikely that this would be achieved with the concentrations contemplated in dental local analgesic cartridges.

Summary

The vasoconstrictors have been responsible for greatly enhancing the effectiveness of the analgesic solutions used by the dental surgeon. These vasoconstrictors are used in extremely small amounts and have minimal disadvantages unless there are complications due to interaction with other drugs as mentioned in Chapter 7. The most common vasoconstrictor to be used in Great Britain is adrenaline, although felypressin is usually used when prilocaine is the local anaesthetic drug.

It seems likely that pharmacological research will be directed towards discovering a new local analgesic drug which also has vasoconstrictor activity, thus doing away with the need for the addition of a vasoconstrictor to the analgesic solution. From the practical viewpoint, if the dental surgeon wants prolonged analgesia, then 2 per cent lignocaine with 1 : 80 000 adrenaline could be used; for a shorter period, 3 per cent prilocaine with 0·03 iu/ml felypressin; and for the shortest period then a local analgesic without vasoconstrictor. In this respect, either prilocaine or especially mepivacaine used without constrictors will provide longer analgesia than lignocaine on its own as lignocaine has no vasoconstrictive action on terminal arterioles.

REVERSING ANAESTHESIA

After a patient has had dental treatment under local anaesthesia, there is a period during which the numbness of the soft tissues persists. Occasionally this may be a nuisance, for example, when the lips and the tongue are numb and the person wishes to dine or when a wind-instrument player wants to perform. With this in mind, attempts have been made to discover methods of reversing the soft-tissue numbness induced by dental local anaesthetic drugs.

In 1985, Dr S. R. Watt-Smith reported his preliminary findings to the meeting of the British Society for Dental Research. Using a solution of the alpha-adrenoceptor drug phentolamine, he had been able to reverse the numbness from local anaesthesia when solutions of lignocaine with adrenaline or mepivacaine with adrenaline had been used. The reversal was achieved by phentolamine abolishing the vasoconstriction induced by the adrenaline. Phentolamine was inactive against the numbness produced by prilocaine with felypressin.

In his experiments, a patient received a routine injection of either lignocaine with adrenaline or mepivacaine with adrenaline. This would eliminate pain sensation in the teeth and also produce some associated soft-tissue numbness. Thirty minutes later the injection was repeated in the same site using a solution of 2 mg/ml phentolamine, the volume of solution being half that of the previous injection of standard local anaesthetic solution. For example, if 1 ml of 2 per cent lignocaine with 1 : 80 000 adrenaline had been used, then only 0·5 ml of the phentolamine solution was required. The period of dental analgesia and soft-tissue numbness would then be reduced to about 15 minutes instead of otherwise persisting very much longer, possibly for 2 or 3 hours. The patients were carefully monitored during these experiments and no deleterious effects were found. Dr Watt-Smith is continuing with his research on phentolamine, and it is possible that at a future date other drugs may be found suitable for using to reverse the unwanted effects of local anaesthetic injections.

REFERENCES

Aellig W. H., Laurence D. R., O'Neil R. et al. (1970) Cardiac effects of adrenaline and felypressin as vasoconstrictors in local anaesthesia for oral surgery under diazepam sedation. *Br. J. Anaesth.* **42**, 174.

Baird D. P. and Scott D. B. (1965) The systemic absorption of local anaesthetic drugs. *Br. J. Anaesth.* **37**, 394.

Berling C. (1958) Carbocaine in local anaesthesia in the oral cavity. *Särtr. Odontol. Revy.* **9**, 1.

Berling C. (1966) Octapressin as a vasoconstrictor in dental plexus anaesthesia. *Odontol. Revy.* **17**, 369.

Boakes A. J., Laurence D. R., Lovel K. W. et al. (1972) Adverse reactions to local anaesthetic/vasoconstrictor preparations. *Br. Dent. J.* **133**, 137.

Cannell H., Walters H., Beckett A. H. et al. (1975) Circulating levels of lignocaine after perioral injections. *Br. Dent. J.* **138**, 87.

Cardwell J. E. and Cawson R. A. (1969) A comparison of 2 per cent lignocaine local anesthetic solutions containing adrenaline 1/80 000 and 1/250 000. IADR (British Division), Abstract No. 72.

Galley A. H. (1969) Personal communication.

Goldman V. (1965) Citanest in dental surgery. *Acta Anaesthesiol. Scand.* Suppl. XVI, 297.

Goldman V. (1969) Personal communication.

Goldman V. et al. (1970) A study of the interaction between tricyclic antidepressants and some local anaesthetic solutions containing vasoconstrictors. Proceedings of the 3rd Asian and Australian Congress of Anaesthesiology. *Anaesthesiology* 517–523.

Goldman V. and Evers H. (1969) Prilocaine–felypressin— a new combination for dental analgesia. *Dent. Pract. Dent. Rec.* **19**, 2.

Goldman V., Killey H. C. and Wright C. (1966) Effects of local analgesic agents and vasoconstrictors on rabbit's ears. *Acta Anaesthesiol. Scand.* Suppl. XXIII, 353.

Kaliciak H. A. and Chan C. C. (1986) Distribution of prilocaine in body fluids and tissues in lethal overdose. *J. Analyt. Toxicol.* **10**, 75.

Lambrianidis T., Rood J. P. and Sowray J. H. (1980) Dental analgesia by jet injection. *Br. J. Oral Surg.* **17**, 227.

Ludwig S. C. (1981) Acute toxic methemoglobinemia following dental analgesia. *Ann. Emerg. Med.* **10**, 265.

Mongar J. L. (1955) A study of two methods of testing local anaesthetics in man. *Br. J. Pharmacol. Chemother.* **10**, 240.

Moore A. M. and Dunsky J. L. (1983) Bupivacaine anesthesia—a clinical trial for endodontic therapy. *Oral Surg.* **55**, 176.

Oliver L. P. (1974) Local anaesthesia—a review of practice. *Aust. Dent. J.* **19**, 313.

Persson G. (1971) Ornithine–vasopressin (POR-8) as a vasoconstrictor in anaesthetics used for ordinary dental treatment. *Scand. J. Dent. Res.* **79**, 441.

Rood J. P. (1976) Inferior alveolar nerve blocks, the use of 5 per cent lignocaine. *Br. Dent. J.* **140**, 413.

Ryder W. (1970) The electrocardiogram in dental anaesthesia. *Anaesthesia* **25**, 46.

Sowray J. H. (1986) Local anaesthetics. In: Derrick D. D. (ed.), *The Dental Annual.* Bristol, Wright. pp. 259–269.

Chapter 5

INSTRUMENTS

CHOICE OF EQUIPMENT

There are several considerations to be made prior to selecting a hypodermic syringe for use in the dental surgery.

1. Ease of handling

It is important that the syringe fits comfortably into the hand and that both injection and aspiration may be easily performed using only one hand, as the other is almost invariably required for the retraction of the soft tissues. The less movement of the fingers which is required during injection the better, and it is here that power-operated syringes have an appreciable advantage. For injections using a 30-gauge needle, infiltrations can be accomplished with 14–35 kPa (2–5 lb/in²) pressure and for palatal injections a pressure of 345–3450 kPa (50–500 lb/in²) is required. A force of about 3·5 kg (8 lb) has to be exerted on the plunger

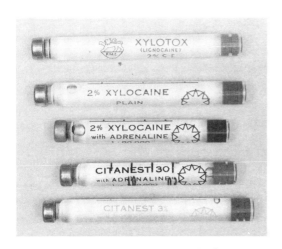

Fig. 5.1. Cartridges of local analgesic.

and piston to produce a pressure of 930 kPa (135 lb/in²) behind the needle, and a 1·8 ml glass cartridge (Cooke-Waite) bursts at about 3450–4140 kPa (500–600 lb/in²) (*Fig.* 5.1).

2. Aspiration

It is absolutely essential that aspiration can be performed with the syringe as many regions of the mouth are highly vascular. Should an intra-vascular injection be given, then—apart from its failing to achieve analgesia—the initial toxicity of the local analgesic is increased many times and this may result in the patient fainting or in more severe untoward effects. After circulating and mixing in the bloodstream, the concentration rapidly becomes diminished.

It is the initial impact of the local analgesic solution on the myocardium which produces a very rapid increase in the heart rate. This may distress the patient and can cause syncope, cardiac arrhythmias and even more severe side-effects, particularly to a patient who has already experienced cardiac damage or has hypertension.

The regions of maximum risk, where aspiration should always be performed, are when administering:

a. Posterior superior dental nerve blocks, when the pterygoid plexus of veins may be entered.

b. Infiltrating, particularly deeply, in the buccal region of the upper second and third molars, and in the palate.

c. Infraorbital nerve blocks.

d. Inferior dental nerve blocks.

e. Mental nerve blocks.

f. All major nerve blocks such as the maxillary and mandibular.

METHODS OF ASPIRATION

Aspiration is achieved by inserting the needle into the tissues to its final position and then creating a negative pressure within the cartridge and thus the lumen of the needle. If a blood vessel has been entered then blood will flow back into the analgesic solution in the cartridge where it will be easily seen.

There are two main ways in which aspiration may be achieved:

1. By retraction of the bung in the cartridge, either manually or by means of a power-operated syringe.

2. By using a special self-aspirating cartridge with a resilient bung.

Whichever of these methods is employed the following are necessary:

a. An airtight seal between the exterior of the needle and the sealing disc of the cartridge which it has perforated.

b. The needle point must be buried completely in the soft tissues, hence a markedly tapered point would need to be inserted to a greater depth than one with a short bevel.

c. The needle should have a sufficiently wide lumen to permit a free flow of blood. It has been recommended that for aspiration the needle should be of not less than 26 or 27 gauge as a thinner lumen will become blocked, especially if the blood is particularly viscous.

1. Retraction of the cartridge bung

To retract the bung it has to be positively connected to the piston of the syringe. This is usually achieved by having a barb, spear or corkscrew spiral type of fitting on the end of the plunger (*Figs.* 5.2, 5.3). An alternative is to use cartridges with tapped inserts in the ends of the bungs so that a threaded end of the syringe plunger can be screwed into them.

To load a syringe using manual retraction of the bung it is easiest to engage the rubber bung with the barb or screw before fitting the needle, otherwise the pressure exerted on the plunger will result in displacement of some of the solution from the cartridge. An alternative technique where a barb is employed is to give the plunger a sudden sharp blow which will result in only minimal loss of analgesic.

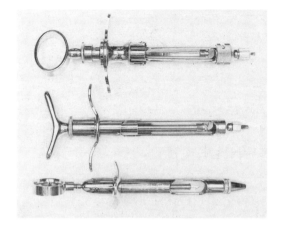

Fig. 5.2. Aspirating syringes. The ring type of handle facilitates the retraction of the plunger for aspiration.

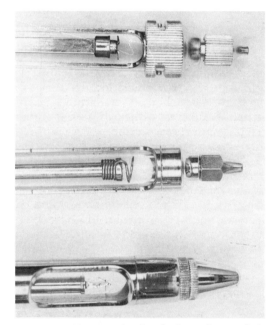

Fig. 5.3. Close-up showing various plunger fittings enabling positive engagement of the bung.

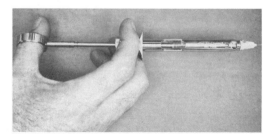

Fig. 5.4. Well-designed metal aspirating syringe with ring handle and finger grip on the barrel.

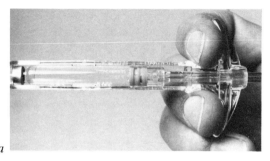 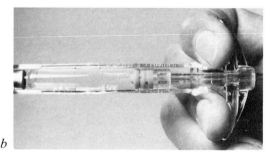

a

b

Fig. 5.5. *a, b,* Resilient bung on the Astra aspirating cartridge showing bulging of the bung when pressure is exerted.

Not only must the barb on the plunger engage the rubber bung but it must be relatively easy to retract the plunger using only one hand, which usually necessitates a ring on the end of the plunger to engage the thumb and a firm finger grip on the body of the syringe (*Fig.* 5.4).

2. The self-aspirating cartridge

Aspiration may be achieved without retraction of the cartridge bung if a special resilient variety, which was advocated by Jorgensen, is employed. When pressure is applied to the rubber diaphragm it bulges into the cartridge chamber, displacing a little of the fluid. When the pressure is released the diaphragm springs back and thus creates a negative pressure within the cartridge and the needle (*Fig.* 5.5). Should the latter be in a blood vessel, then blood will enter the cartridge and be clearly visible (*Fig.* 5.6).

Astra Chemicals Ltd have marketed such a system using a special cartridge with a resilient diaphragm into which fits the modified end of the syringe plunger. At one time the Astra aspirating syringe was available as a prepacked disposable plastic instrument (*Fig.* 5.7). The firm now manufactures a similar metal syringe for use with these cartridges (*Fig.* 5.8), and

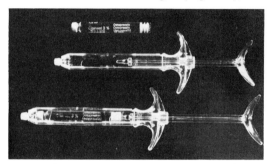

Fig. 5.7. Astra disposable aspirating syringe.

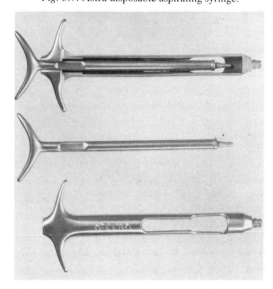

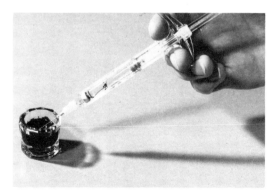

Fig. 5.6. Ink entering the cartridge owing to negative pressure.

Fig. 5.8. The Astra self-aspirating syringe. This syringe is made of an aluminium alloy and should not be immersed in alkalis, sterilization being by dry heat only. Later models are more robust.

the Amalgamated Dental Company markets a metal syringe which can be fitted with a plunger which is also suitable for this form of aspiration.

The only disadvantages of this system are:

a. That a small quantity of the local analgesic solution has to be injected before aspiration can be performed.

b. The amount which may be aspirated is far more limited than with an aspirating syringe system. However, research by Corkery and Barrett (1973) and other workers would indicate that it is completely adequate.

STERILIZATION

As mentioned in Chapter 6, the days of using boiling water for sterilizing surgical instruments have long since passed, the dry heat sterilizer or autoclave being the method of choice for the majority of practices and hospitals. However, whereas autoclaving may be adequate for the vast majority of surgical instruments, it is unsatisfactory for hypodermic needles, hence dental needles must never be reused. The problems encountered in attempting to resterilize fine-gauge needles are these:

a. Organisms may be sealed inside the lumen of the needle by blood which has seeped in after the injection has been given.

b. The blood itself may be infected, as occurs in diseases such as infective hepatitis.

c. Blocking of the needle lumen by blood prevents moist heat reaching organisms, so that sterilization does not occur—considerably higher temperatures being required to achieve complete sterilization by dry heat instead of moist heat.

d. Resistance of the organisms within the lumen may be increased by their being surrounded by blood.

e. Blood and serum may contain pyrogens which cause a pyrexia when a contaminated needle is used to inject another patient.

Disposable needles

An obvious alternative to resterilization is to use a fresh needle for each patient, thus obviating the risk of cross-infection. If this is done, the needles become, in effect, disposable. This means that they can be prepackaged and sterilized at the factory, the commonest and most efficient method being by gamma radiation. Most of these needles have plastic hubs incorporated in their construction, and these are either screwed on to the cartridge syringe or rely upon a friction grip to retain them (*Fig.* 5.9).

The use of the disposable needle brings further advantages. The needle will not be subjected to the trauma of repeated sterilization and hence a far thinner gauge with a finer point may be used (*Fig.* 5.10). Thus the Standards Association of Australia recommend a bevel for disposable needles of 12° instead of either the 18° or 30° which was formerly used. Disposable single-use needles are commonly made in the smaller gauges, 27–30, although they are available in gauges 23–30. The fine gauges, of

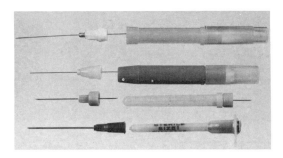

Fig. 5.9. Varieties of prepacked disposable needles and their containers which have been sterilized by gamma radiation.

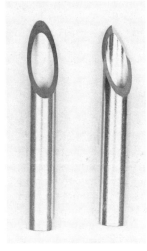

Fig. 5.10. Varieties of needle points.

course, permit easier penetration of the tissues and thus far less discomfort for the patient. Also they are essential for intraligamentary injections where a very fine gauge is needed because the periodontal membrane is such a thin fibrous layer with restricted access.

The disadvantage of fine needles when used for regional block injections in particular, is that they appear to penetrate blood vessels far more easily and thus the risk of bleeding into the soft tissues may be increased. Killey and Kay (1967) consider that this is possibly the cause of trismus following the administration of inferior dental injections with very fine gauge needles, as mentioned on page 152. Furthermore, as the needles penetrate blood vessels more easily, then there is an increased chance of giving an intravascular injection.

Disposable needle–cartridge units

A logical development from the disposable needle is the disposable needle–cartridge unit, such as the Disposall unit which at one time was marketed by the Pharmaceutical Manufacturing Company (*Fig.* 5.11).

This eliminates any risk of the solution being contaminated during loading when the needle pierces the rubber diaphragm, as the needle and cartridge are integral with each other and thus sterilized after they are joined.

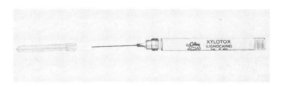

Fig. 5.11. The Disposall dental cartridge unit.

Dufar Cartrix System

A more recent disposable needle–cartridge unit is the Dufar Cartrix System (*Fig.* 5.12). The advantage of this is that the solution only comes into contact with the needle when pressure is applied to the bung and the thin rubber diaphragm breaks (*Fig.* 5.13), thus guaranteeing sterility and avoiding any chance of damage to or blocking of the needle.

A special syringe has been designed to

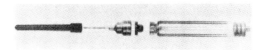

Fig. 5.12. The components of the Dufar Cartrix System.

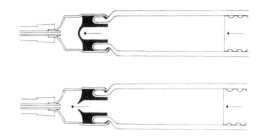

Fig. 5.13. The thin rubber diaphragm breaks when pressure is applied to the bung in the Dufar Cartrix System.

accommodate this unit. It employs a split barrel which is held together by a circlip after insertion of the cartridge (*Fig.* 5.14). This has a threaded bung (*Fig.* 5.15) on to which the plunger is screwed to permit aspiration.

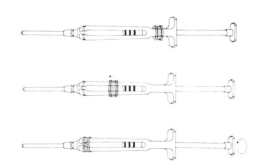

Fig. 5.14. Assembling the special syringe in the Dufar Cartrix System.

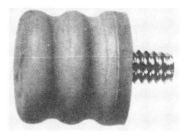

Fig. 5.15. Threaded bung of the Dufar Cartrix System.

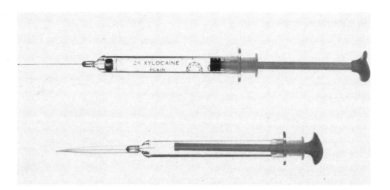

Fig. 5.16. Disposable syringe which was marketed by the Pharmaceutical Manufacturing Company.

SYRINGES

Fully disposable syringes

A further advance was made when the Pharmaceutical Manufacturing Company produced their fully disposable syringe with needle already attached (*Fig.* 5.16). Unfortunately, however, the syringe was somewhat clumsy to use, as the plastic components did not run smoothly and it had to be loaded with a cartridge, which again introduced the risk of infection.

As stated earlier, Astra Chemicals Ltd marketed a fully disposable plastic syringe which employed their aspirating cartridges (*Fig.* 5.7). The syringe came in a plastic sterilized bag, but unfortunately a needle and the cartridge had to be fitted to it prior to use, thus introducing the risk, albeit slight, of infection. It has been replaced by a metal model (*Fig.* 5.8).

Ideally, a disposable syringe should come ready loaded with the local analgesic solution. For some years, certain drugs have been marketed in sterile, ready-loaded syringes complete with needle (*Fig.* 5.17). A more recent addition to this range has been the introduction of Xylocard (*Fig.* 5.18), which is a sterile loaded syringe containing 5 ml of plain 2 per cent lignocaine for treatment of ventricular tachyarrhythmias. It would seem a logical step for dental local analgesics to be similarly packaged.

Prior to the manufacture of cartridges of analgesic solution, glass and metal or all-metal syringes were used and the solution was drawn up into the barrel of the syringe by withdrawing the plunger. It is possible that some of these

a

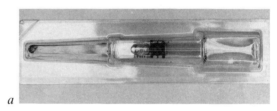

b

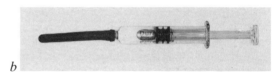

Fig. 5.17. *a, b,* A disposable syringe ready loaded with an anabolic drug, Durabolin.

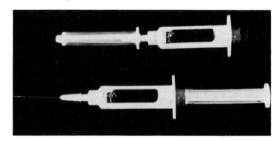

Fig. 5.18. Xylocard, a disposable syringe ready loaded with lignocaine. The protective needle guard becomes the plunger of the syringe by being screwed into a threaded cartridge bung.

syringes are still in use. The hypodermic or hypomucosal syringe of this type with a glass barrel had the advantage that aspiration could be performed by withdrawing the piston immediately prior to injecting. Blood was readily visible as a contaminant of the analgesic solution when a vessel had been entered.

The non-disposable cartridge syringe

The metal cartridge syringe (*Fig.* 5.19) is extremely simple to prepare for use, as the analgesic solution is prepacked in a sterile state within a disposable cartridge (*Fig.* 5.1). It is probably the most commonly used type and is designed to take a cartridge containing 1·5, 1·8, 2 or 2·2 ml of solution. The cartridge has a depressible rubber bung serving as a piston at one end, with a thin metal or rubber sealing disc at the other, the glass tube of the cartridge taking the place of the barrel of the syringe. The syringe uses a hollow needle which has a sharp cutting point at both ends and, when the cartridge is loaded into the syringe, the sealing disc is perforated by the end of the needle which projects inside the syringe. Movement of the plunger forces the rubber bung along the lumen of the cartridge and thus the solution is discharged via the needle.

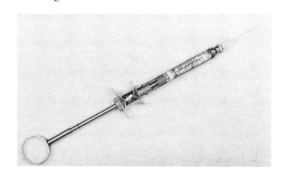

Fig. 5.19. Side-loading aspirating cartridge fitted with disposable needle.

There are two main ways of loading a metal cartridge syringe (*Fig.* 5.20).

1. The breech-loading type is hinged so that the handle and piston are moved to display the opening in the end of the barrel through which the cartridge is inserted, and when the cartridge is in place then the barrel and piston are brought back into alignment.

2. The ejector or side-loading type has no hinge but instead has an opening along one side of the barrel through which the cartridge is inserted. This design also incorporates, at the piston end of the barrel, a spring which is compressed when the cartridge is in place, thus retaining it.

The metal cartridge syringe retains its disposable needle by means of a plastic hub which

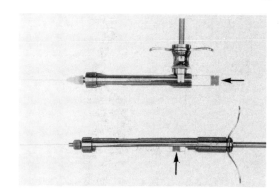

Fig. 5.20. Syringes may be loaded in different ways. The 'breech-loading' syringe (*top*). The 'ejector' or 'side-loading' type (*bottom*). Arrows indicate the direction of insertion of the cartridge.

is an integral part of the needle. The old-fashioned reusable-type needle was retained by means of a separate metal hub which slid over the needle and then screwed on to the barrel. Although the reusable needle should never be used on more than one patient, it has the advantage that its length and angulation may be varied by using different hubs (*Fig.* 5.21). For injections with a reusable-type needle, a long hub may be fitted to give additional support during papillary injections, and a curved one to bend the needle into a more convenient position for posterior superior dental injections and maxillary nerve blocks.

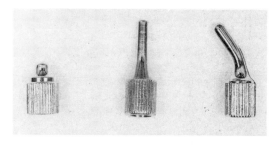

Fig. 5.21. Varieties of needle hub for the all-metal cartridge syringe.

Aspirating syringes

Shown in *Fig.* 5.2 are three syringes with various methods of engaging the rubber bung, and, while theoretically all three may be used as aspirating syringes, in practice the middle one could not be employed as it would require two hands to operate, one to hold the barrel of the syringe and the other to retract the plunger. With an aspirating syringe it is essential that the barrel can be firmly grasped with the fingers, and the plunger retracted with the thumb of the same hand as, with the vast majority of dental injections it is impractical to use two hands to control the syringe (*Fig.* 5.4).

The latest syringe marketed by the Amalgamated Dental Company incorporates alternative plungers so that aspiration may be achieved by either manual retraction of the bung or the use of an aspirating cartridge (*Fig.* 5.22).

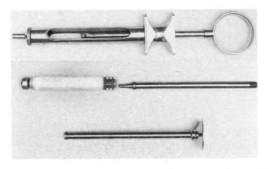

Fig. 5.22. Amalgamated Dental Company syringe with choice of plungers. The top syringe has a twisted barbed end for aspiration, the middle one has an Astra aspirating type and the bottom syringe has a non-aspirating pattern.

Power-operated syringes

The advantages of power-operated syringes are several:

a. They provide constant pressure and thus tend to give a smoother injection.

b. Only minimal movement of the hand is required when giving the injection, so that it is more comfortable for the operator and the syringe is more easily controlled.

c. The operator's hand is less visible to the patient, as described above.

d. The syringes usually incorporate aspiration.

1. Spring-driven syringe

The Hypomat (*Fig.* 5.23), manufactured by Medivance Products Ltd, uses an oil-dampened spring to provide smooth actuation. To prepare the syringe for use, the spring is compressed

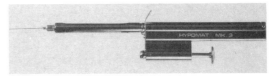

a

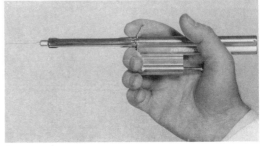

b

Fig. 5.23. *a, b,* The Hypomat Mk 3 spring-actuated aspirating syringe.

against a plastic stand which is grooved to protect the aspirating hook from damage (*Fig.* 5.24). The single plunger permits both injection and aspiration and has an extremely effective action. The syringe employs conventional dental cartridges and the speed of injection may be very accurately controlled by varying the pressure on the plunger. It is available with different strengths of spring.

Shown in *Fig.* 5.25 is a regional nerve block being given with three different syringes. With the conventional dental syringe, it can be seen that the finger travel necessary during injection will be considerable and there is obviously no way in which the plunger can be retracted. With the aspirating syringe, aspiration can be performed, because the barb on the plunger engages the cartridge bung. However, the plunger travel is long and the patient can actually see and be apprehensive of the plunger being depressed. With the Hypomat, hand movement on the plunger for both injection and aspiration is minimal and the patient cannot easily see when the injection is being given.

2. Gas-actuated syringe

An alternative power-operated syringe was the Densco S.220 (*Figs.* 5.26, 5.27), the force for

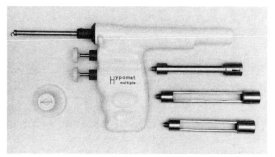

a

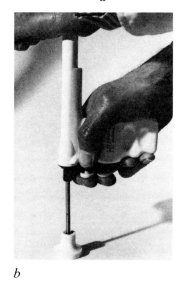

b

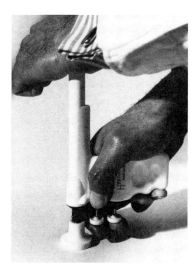

c

Fig. 5.24. *a,* The Hypomat Mk 2 syringe kit showing the former pistol-type design. The circular plastic stand used for compressing the spring may be seen on the left of the illustration. *b, c,* The spring being compressed. This Mk 2 Hypomat had one trigger or button for aspiration and one for injection.

injection being provided by the vaporization of a liquid fluorocarbon known as Freon. Although this particular instrument has been discontinued, the principle may be reapplied on future syringes. Several types of Freon exist; one example is Freon 22 (monochlorodifluoromethane, $CHClF_2$), which boils at 5 °C to produce a pressure of 932 kPa (135 lb/in^2) at normal room temperature 24·5 °C. Two drops of this solution produced enough energy by vaporization to inject 1·8 ml at a pressure of over 690 kPa (100 lb/in^2).

These fluorocarbons are colourless, almost odourless, non-inflammable and virtually non-toxic. The Freon was put in a hermetically sealed cartridge which contained enough gas for 50 injections at a rate of injection of 1 ml in about 15 seconds. The Freon cartridge was sterilized by cold sterilization, but the rest of the syringe could be autoclaved.

The syringe was used with a pen grasp for accuracy during needle insertion and this grip did not need to be changed before injection, which was given very smoothly because pressure on the plunger was evenly applied. The instrument provided limited automatic aspiration before each injection. The plunger was re-compressed by using either of the plastic tools provided, one being used as with the Hypomat (*Fig.* 5.24) and the other as shown in *Fig.* 5.28.

At one stage it was anticipated that the syringe would be modified to run off compressed air, when it could easily become an integral part of the dental unit. However, this has not yet come to pass and the production of the S.220 has been discontinued.

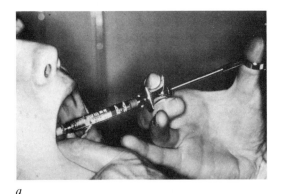

a

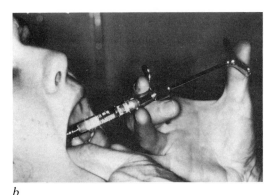

b

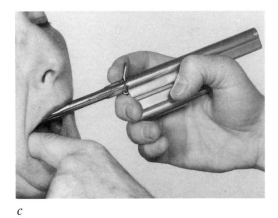

c

Fig. 5.25. *a*, Regional nerve block being given with conventional syringe. *b*, Metal aspirating syringe in use. *c*, Hypomat Mk 3.

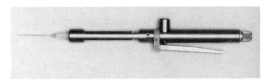

Fig. 5.26. Densco S.220 gas-actuated syringe ready for use.

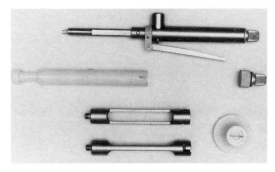

Fig. 5.27. Densco S.220 syringe kit.

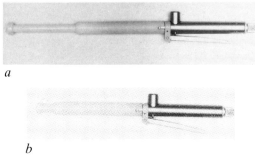

a

b

Fig. 5.28. *a*, *b*, Plunger of Densco S.220 being 'recompressed' using a plastic tool.

Intraligamentary syringes

These are specially designed for injecting very small doses of local anaesthetic solution into the periodontal membrane. Because this structure is so thin, a very fine gauge needle such as 30 gauge is used.

There are two main patterns, one is a pen-type with lever actuation and the other is a pistol-type with trigger actuation. The instrument needs to feel comfortable when used because the intraligamentary injection requires precision for achieving successful analgesia. Access at the back of the mouth may be difficult to obtain without bending the needle and hence a syringe with an angled nozzle may be advantageous. As a principle, it is very undesirable for syringe needles to be bent as this weakens the metal and makes breakage more likely. However, the intraligamentary injection needs to be given accurately, and in some cases this will necessitate the needle being carefully bent. Fortunately, the needle is only inserted a very short distance into the tissues so breakage is much less likely than with most other injection techniques.

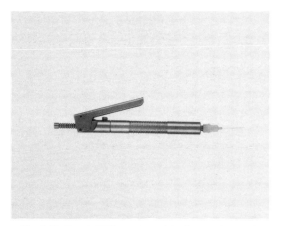

Fig. 5.29. Ever's PDL pen-type intraligamentary syringe with all-metal barrel containing the anaesthetic cartridge. This is a well-made reliable instrument.

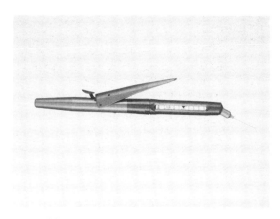

Fig. 5.30. Citoject intraligamentary syringe with an angled nozzle for ease of access. The cartridge remains visible and is protected by a clear plastic sleeve.

Examples of intraligamentary syringes are shown in *Figs.* 5.29–5.33. *Fig.* 5.29 shows a typical pen-type, *Fig.* 5.30 the pen-type with angled nozzle, and *Figs.* 5.31–5.33 pistol-grip types. The Intra-lig syringe (*Fig.* 5.33) is shown with the pistol-type handle, but this may be readily modified, as the pistol handle can be removed and the syringe converted into the pen-type with lever actuation.

Most of these syringes deliver between 0·15 and 0·2 ml with each dose. Sometimes the injection pressure may be quite high as a fine needle is being used and the injection site is in firm tissue confined between the hard tissues of bone on one side and tooth root on the other. The glass cartridge breaks at a pressure of about 3450–4140 kPa (500–600 lb/in^2), and it has been recorded that a palatal infiltration injection—another site where the injection pressure may be high—sometimes produces a pressure of up to about 3450 kPa (500 lb/in^2). Because of this slight risk of the cartridge glass breaking, it is prudent to use an intraligamental syringe where the cartridge is protected. Many of these syringes have metal barrels but the Ligmaject and Citoject syringes have the advantage of clear plastic sleeves so that the columns of the solution remaining in the cartridges may be seen. With most of the other all-metal barrelled syringes, an estimate of the amount of anaesthetic fluid remaining within the cartridge may be assessed by noting how much of the metal rod projecting at the back of the syringe is visible.

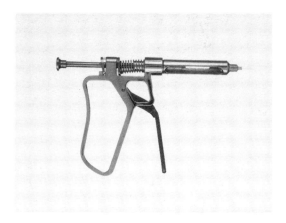

Fig. 5.31. Ligmaject intraligamentary syringe with pistol-type handle. The cartridge remains visible and is protected by a clear plastic sleeve.

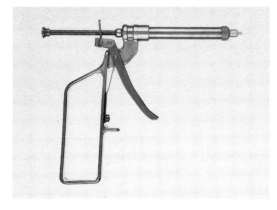

Fig. 5.32. Peripress intraligmentary syringe with all-metal barrel.

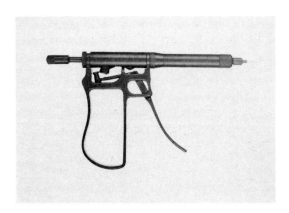

Fig. 5.33. Intra-lig intraligamentary syringe shown with a pistol-type handle. This syringe may be readily modified to become a pen-type model.

JET INJECTION

The concept of jet injection as a method of administering local analgesics probably arose from the accidental injection of grease into the tissues by engineers using compressed-air grease-guns for lubricating purposes. A mechanical engineer called Sutermeister reported that men employed by the US railways sometimes developed abscesses which arose from deposits of grease deep in the tissues. It was also noticed that mechanics servicing motor vehicles who received severe injuries due to the misuse of high-pressure grease-guns did not seem to feel pain at the time of the injection. The damage to the tissues which resulted from these accidents probably arose from the infected material which had been injected and not from the actual method of introduction.

Medical jet injectors

In 1947 a compressed-air jet injector for medical use, called the Hypospray, was evaluated and it was found that most patients felt less pain than that caused by a 26-gauge hypodermic needle. It was noted that this instrument was particularly successful with children who regarded it as a spray rather than a syringe.

This jet injector was a single-dose instrument primarily designed for injecting local analgesic solution through the skin. It was a hand-cocked, spring-loaded design and a little later automatic

types such as the Presso-jet and Hypospray Model K were developed. These instruments, which resembled pistols, were electrically powered and able to administer about 500 injections per hour. They are ideal for tasks such as mass inoculations (*Fig.* 5.34), but were not designed for dental use.

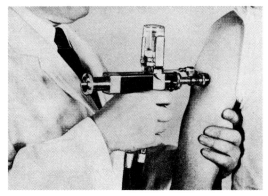

Fig. 5.34. Medical jet injector inoculating a patient.

Dental jet injectors

Dermojet

In 1960 the Dermojet was developed in France for the purpose of depositing a bleb of local analgesic intradermally to produce a weal on the skin or mucosa into which an injection could be performed painlessly. The Dermojet expelled about 0·04 ml of solution with each dose, and its aim was not to produce deep analgesia of the tissues but to provide an adjuvant to the more usual methods of injection.

Panjet

A later development of the Dermojet is the Panjet (*Fig.* 5.35*a*). This is a very similar instrument in its external appearance, but the interior of the instrument has been redesigned and it is quieter in operation. It has a 5 ml glass chamber into which the analgesic solution is loaded and is primed by compressing a spring (*Fig.* 5.35*b*). When the release button is depressed, the Panjet emits analgesic solution in the form of a fine spray which penetrates the surface of the oral mucosa to a depth of 2–6 mm (*Fig.* 5.36).

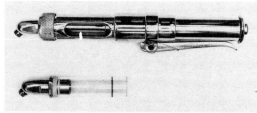

a

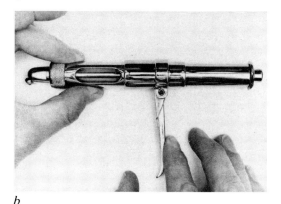

b

Fig. 5.35. *a, b,* The Panjet showing the method of compressing the spring. When the spring is compressed, the release button protrudes from the end of the barrel.

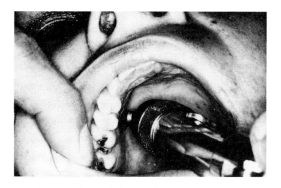

Fig. 5.36. Panjet being used on palatal mucosa.

Main (1967) has recommended that when the Panjet is used for buccal and labial analgesia of the gingivae, the weal should be raised on the attached gingiva and not on the more mobile alveolar mucosa. The jet injector is also of value in obtaining a localized region of analgesia for techniques such as taking subgingival impressions, thus obviating the need for a hypodermic injection. Work by Lambrianidis et al. (1980) suggests that jet injection with more concentrated analgesic solutions may permit jet-injection techniques to replace the ordinary hypodermic injections for many aspects of dental treatment.

Stephens' jet injector

In about 1964 a prototype multiple-dose dental jet injector was constructed by the Amalgamated Dental Engineering Company to the design of R. R. Stephens (*Fig.* 5.37). This instrument was worked by compressed air producing a pressure of up to $20\,700\,\mathrm{kPa}$ ($3000\,\mathrm{lb/in^2}$), and even at low pressure the diameter of its jet was about one-sixth that of a

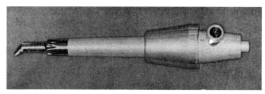

a

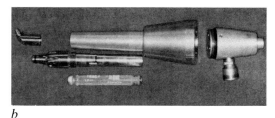

b

Fig. 5.37. *a, b,* The Stephens' jet injector.

26-gauge needle as normally used for infiltration injections. The force exerted by the jet is very small because, although the solution pressure might be up to $20\,700\,\mathrm{kPa}$ ($3000\,\mathrm{lb/in^2}$), the area of the nozzle orifice is only $0.000007\,\mathrm{in^2}$ and therefore the force in this example would be only approximately $\frac{1}{3}\,\mathrm{oz}$. This prototype instrument could inject a dosage of local analgesic solution varying from 0.05 to 0.5 ml, and the loss of sensation produced was equivalent to that expected from a needle injection of the same amount of solution.

Med-E-Jet

This jet injector is powered by a small cartridge of carbon dioxide gas which is contained within the hollow pistol-type handle (*Fig.* 5.38). The

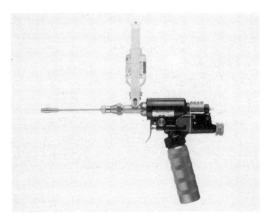

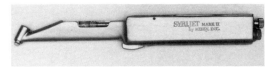

Fig. 5.39. Mizzy Syrijet, Mk 2.

Fig. 5.38. Med-E-Jet jet injector.

local anaesthetic solution is supplied to the syringe via a multi-dose bottle situated above the barrel and this tends to make the instrument look unsightly. Aesthetically, the instrument leaves a lot to be desired, but it does have a major advantage in being the only dental jet injector which will inject as much as 1 ml as a single dose. The volume of solution injected at a single firing may be varied from about 0·2 ml up to 1 ml. With the larger volumes, the solution penetrates deeply into the soft tissues and regional blocks have been administered successfully using this instrument.

Mizzy Syrijet

Another recent jet injector to be marketed for dental use is the Mizzy Syrijet (*Fig.* 5.39). This

has several advantages over its forerunners. It employs cartridges (*Fig.* 5.40), thus facilitating sterility, and the dosage may be varied between 0·05 and 0·2 ml by means of a regulating cylinder at the rear of the gun (*Fig.* 5.41), which is extruded after the gun is cocked (*Fig.* 5.42). The gun is quiet in operation and the trigger actuation is light. The diameter of the jet fired is appreciably less than that of a 30-gauge needle, which accounts for the ready passage of the analgesic into the tissues. The injection site should normally be on attached tissue, otherwise when the jet injector is fired the mucosa

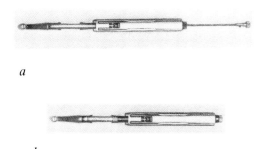

a

b

Fig. 5.40. *a, b,* Mizzy Syrijet being loaded with a local anaesthetic cartridge.

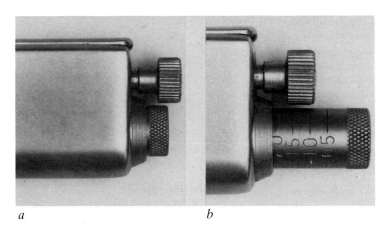

a   *b*

Fig. 5.41. *a, b,* Dose adjustment on the Syrijet.

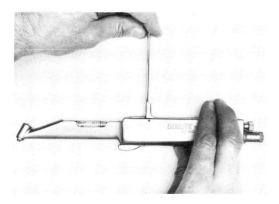

Fig. 5.42. Compressing the spring in the Syrijet.

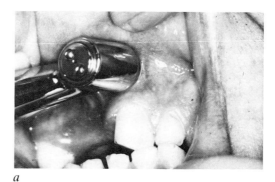

a

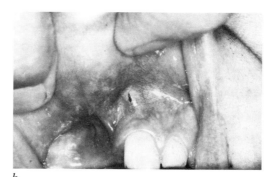

b

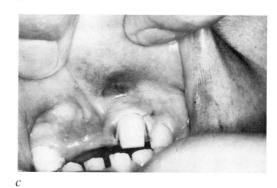

c

Fig. 5.43. a, Syrijet in use, b, Site of injection immediately after using injector. c, Site of injection showing minimal bruising 2 hours later.

will move and this will result in it being traumatized. Likewise, if the instrument is moved during firing the jet will act like a scalpel and cut the tissues (Fig. 14.13).

No pain is normally felt during injection, and if the dosage is low there is little postoperative trauma; however, if maximum dosage is used, as is required for instance for pulpal analgesia, then bruising may occur, but is not normally painful. Fig. 5.43 shows the tissues approximately 2 hours after an injection of 0·4 ml. The difficulty with jet injectors is that if one injects into attached tissues they can only absorb a limited amount of local analgesic without damage, whereas if one fires into unattached tissues they will be cut.

It must be remembered that the solution rapidly diffuses laterally in the tissue planes and therefore no great depth of penetration is achieved. Thus the usual jet injection techniques with very small volumes are of little use for regional nerve blocks and, indeed, even for infiltration injections for pulpal analgesia a conventional syringe is at present to be preferred. However, for the removal of loose teeth or roots and other minor soft-tissue surgery and for palatal analgesia where the insertion of a needle may be painful, the jet injector will prove extremely valuable.

To summarize, the choice of syringe for the majority of dental uses would now seem to lie between the following:

1. The conventional manually operated aspirating syringe, ideally employing an integral needle cartridge unit.
2. A fully disposable syringe which, to provide perfect sterility, should be ready loaded and should also incorporate aspiration.
3. A power-operated syringe, of which the Hypomat is currently the best.

The choice between these three will depend on the personal preference of the operator, and possibly economic considerations.

In addition, it would be desirable for the operator to have an intraligamental syringe as this injection is sometimes most useful. The selection of a suitable syringe should be one which can be used with both 1·8 ml and 2·2 ml cartridges so that there is no restriction on the choice of local anaesthetic solution.

REFERENCES AND FURTHER READING

Alling C. C. and Christopher A. (1974) Status report on dental anesthetic needles and syringes. Report of Councils and Bureaus. *J. Am. Dent. Assoc.* **89,** 1171.

Australian Standard 1264 (1972) *Dental Single-use Cartridge Hypodermic Needles (Sterile).* North Sydney, NSW, Standards Association of Australia.

Australian Standard 1592 (1974) *Dental Hypodermic Needles (Re-usable).* North Sydney, NSW, Standards Association of Australia.

Candy C. T. (1965) The gas-actuated syringe. *N.Z. Dent. J.* 180.

Corkery P. F. and Barrett B. E. (1973) Aspiration using local anaesthetic cartridges with an elastic recoil diaphragm. *J. Dent.* **2,** 72.

Cowan A. (1972) A new aspirating syringe. *Br. Dent. J.* **133,** 547.

El Geneidy A. K., Bloom A. A., Skerman J. H. et al. (1974) Tissue reaction to jet injection. *Oral Surg.* **38,** 501.

Epstein S. (1971) Pressure injection of local anaesthetics: clinical evaluation of an instrument. *J. Am. Dent. Assoc.* **82,** 374.

Lambrianidis T., Rood J. P. and Sowray J. H. (1980) Dental analgesia by jet injection. *Br. J. Oral Surg.* **17,** 227.

Main D. M. G. (1967) Jet injection. *Dent. News* **4,** 7.

Oliver L. P. (1974) Local anaesthesia—a review of practice. *Aust. Dent. J.* **19,** 5.

Rood J. P. (1985) Aspiration in dental local analgesia. In: Derrick D. D. (ed.), *The Dental Annual.* Bristol, Wright, pp. 152–157.

Rood J. P. (1974) The efficiency of a new aspirating system. *J. Dent.* **2,** 18.

Sowray J. H. (1981) Recent advances in jet injection. *Int. J. Oral Surg.* **10,** Suppl. 1, 143.

Stephens R. R. and Kramer I. R. H. (1964) Intra-oral injections by high pressure jet. *Br. Dent. J.* **117,** 465.

Whitehead F. I. H. and Young I. (1968) An intraoral jet injection instrument. *Br. Dent. J.* **125,** 437.

Chapter 6

STERILIZATION AND DISINFECTION

Sterilization is a process which eliminates all living micro-organisms. In dentistry it is essential for syringes and instruments to be sterile prior to use, otherwise they may give rise to serious infection. When an injection is given, the needle is inserted deeply into the tissues and, if infection is present at the site of injection, the forcing of local anaesthetic solution through the tissues will tend to spread it.

Disinfection is a process which eliminates infection due to vegetative organisms, but spores may survive. Thus disinfection is not necessarily as safe a procedure as sterilization. The main methods of sterilization and disinfection are physical methods such as heat and irradiation, or chemical means.

PHYSICAL METHODS

1. Heat

Moist heat

Although boiling water kills most vegetative bacteria within 2 or 3 minutes, bacterial spores and viruses may survive boiling even after many hours. For this reason, the so-called electric 'sterilizer', which formerly was used to boil water continuously, should never be used. The word 'sterilizer' was a misnomer as sterilization did not occur.

The use of the autoclave or pressure-steam sterilizer is the commonest method employed in hospitals in this country and it is also used in some dental surgeries (*Fig.* 6.1). It works on the basis of a pressure cooker and is extremely efficient, provided that the metal drums containing dirty instruments are not overpacked so that the steam is unable to penetrate the load. If a small autoclave is being used, then the instruments should be placed on open shelves.

Tests should be carried out routinely to check that sterilization is adequate and this may be done with chemical indicators such as Browne's tubes, by Bowie's autoclave tape test, by using a standard test pack containing a thermocouple or by using standardized spore papers. Some of these tests are very specialized and care needs to be taken to obtain reliable results. In order to remove air which forms an insulating barrier between the instruments and the steam, the autoclave may have a vacuum extractor or

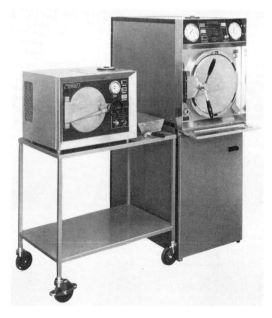

Fig. 6.1. Autoclaves. (Reproduced by courtesy of Surgical Equipment Supplies Ltd.)

devices for eliminating air by displacement—as air is heavier than steam and can be bled off from the bottom of the autoclave—or by creating turbulence.

The recommendations of the Medical Research Council Working Party are that autoclaving times for actual exposure to steam after the steam has penetrated the load are:

> 3 minutes at 134 °C
> 10 minutes at 126 °C
> 15 minutes at 121 °C

The steam is at a pressure of about 104–207 kPa (15–30 lb/in²). If these conditions are met then the autoclave will destroy all organisms and spores to give complete sterilization (*Fig.* 6.2).

Dry heat

Dry heat is only effective on scrupulously clean instruments as proteinaceous material, such as may be left from dried serum, will protect

viruses and some bacteria. Ideally, sterilization should be done by autoclaving, especially of instruments which may have been contaminated with organisms such as the Hepatitis B virus.

The hot-air sterilizer is a popular method of sterilization used in general dental practice and hospitals (*Fig.* 6.3). It is more convenient than moist heat methods as steam does not condense in the surgery and also instruments are less likely to corrode and do not require drying after sterilization. The disadvantages of this method are that in dry conditions organisms are much harder to kill than when they are wet, also dry heat has very little power of penetration, and unless very high temperatures are used the method is slow (*see Fig.* 6.2). The instruments also need a considerable time to cool after sterilization and the temper of metal instruments may be lost. Care must be taken to avoid putting an instrument containing 'soft' solder in a hot-air sterilizer at too high a temperature or the solder will melt.

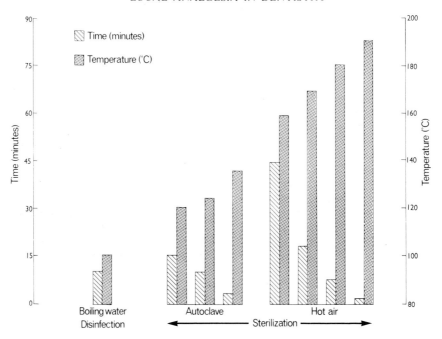

LOCAL ANALGESIA IN DENTISTRY

Fig. 6.2. Histogram showing the relative efficiency of the various methods of sterilization.

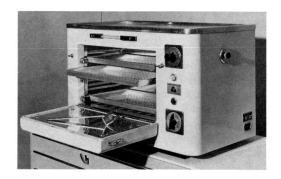

Fig. 6.3. Hot-air sterilizer. (Reproduced by courtesy of the Wright Dental Group.)

Sterilization is achieved by dry heat at:

160 °C for 45 minutes
170 °C for 15 minutes
180 °C for 7½ minutes
190 °C for 1½ minutes

These exposure times are considered to be sufficient to kill all spores. As they are the times for which the high temperature should be maintained, that is the 'holding times', the actual sterilization cycle is twice as long.

In many hot-air ovens the space heating is very irregular so that overheating may occur in one part of the oven, yet in another part the temperature may not rise high enough to sterilize. Because of this it is advisable to assume that, for example, an oven temperature of 160 °C for 1 hour should be used for sterilization, as this will probably result in the recommended minimum period of 45 minutes at 160 °C being achieved. If a hot-air sterilizer is used in general dental practice then very great care should be taken not to open the sterilizer during the sterilization cycle, as such actions as adding new instruments lower the temperature and may mix dirty and sterile instruments.

Flaming

Some small metal instruments may be sterilized by this method, but is has the disadvantage that the temper of the metal may be spoilt by overheating as it is difficult to assess what temperature has been reached. This method is of no use for hypodermic needles as they would be ruined by the excessive heat needed.

2. Irradiation

This is a relatively new method of sterilization and has excellent penetrating power which permits the sterilization of an instrument contained within a pack. It is a method which is being used for sterilizing disposable needles and syringes.

The dosage used for sterilization is about 2·5 megarads and the irradiation is obtained from gamma rays emitted from radioactive material such as cobalt-60, or from beta particles from a linear accelerator. As may be imagined, this method of sterilization is complex and therefore only feasible in large establishments.

CHEMICAL METHODS

These methods involve the use of liquid or gaseous compounds.

1. Liquid disinfectants

Generally the liquids are very unreliable for achieving sterility as they do not kill viruses and both vegetative and sporing bacteria may survive so that liquids tend to disinfect rather than sterilize. Another snag is that these liquids may not penetrate sufficiently to achieve destruction of bacteria harbouring in the crevices of instruments, and some liquids are inactivated by organic materials such as serum and pus.

According to the HMSO publication *The Use of Chemical Disinfectants in Hospitals* (Kelsey and Maurer, 1972), there are four main indications for the use of disinfectants:

a. The cleansing of skin and mucous membranes.
b. The disinfection of instruments when physical methods are unsuitable.
c. Making potentially infected or dirty articles safe for subsequent handling.
d. Decontamination of surfaces such as walls and floors.

The chemical disinfectants have been subdivided into the following groups:

i. Phenolics such as Izal, Dettol and Jeyes Fluid. All the phenolics are compatible with anionic and non-ionic detergents.

ii. Alcohols, often used with other agents such as chlorhexidine and iodine. The alcohols have a wide range of antibacterial action and are rapid. Absolute alcohol is not as efficient as 70 per cent ethyl alcohol.

iii. Halogens such as hypochlorite solution and iodine solution. These are compatible with anionic and non-ionic detergents. They have a wide range of antibacterial activity, except for *Mycobacterium tuberculosis*.

iv. Aldehydes such as formalin solution.

v. Quaternary ammonium compounds such as cetrimide. All of these are incompatible with anionic detergents and they have a narrow range of antibacterial activity.

vi. Pine fluids such as Zal. These are good deodorants but have little disinfectant activity.

2. Gases

Ethylene oxide gas (C_2H_4O) is useful for sterilizing heat-sensitive materials. It has good penetrating powers and destroys all bacteria including spores, but unfortunately it is flammable. Although this process needs relatively complex apparatus, it is used in some hospitals for sterilizing dental instruments.

Formaldehyde gas kills bacteria and paraformaldehyde tablets will slowly disintegrate to release this gas. Because of this process, an instrument cabinet may be disinfected by placing paraformaldehyde tablets within it. This is an unreliable method as the vapour has poor powers of penetration and is difficult to control.

PROBLEMS OF STERILIZATION IN LOCAL ANALGESIA

The mouth contains a profuse flora of bacteria and micro-organisms and there is a risk of the syringe needle transferring organisms from the surface of the oral mucosa deep into the tissues when an injection is given. Except for those patients with a lowered resistance, this is probably quite a small risk as the body has inherent defence mechanisms against infection and an organism transferred into the tissues in this way would probably be destroyed quickly by circulating antibodies in the bloodstream. It is unusual to see patients with evidence of soft-tissue infection following an injection of local

analgesic, although Barnard in 1976 reported two cases of extensive osteomyelitis of the jaws as a possible sequel to local anaesthetic injections. Thus the risk of infection exists and it may be minimized by drying the mucosa and applying an antiseptic solution, such as 2 per cent chlorhexidine digluconate (Hibitane) in alcohol or tincture of iodine, prior to injection. It has been said that iodine corrodes stainless steel, but if a needle of this type is used for the injection there will be minimal time for the iodine on the mucosa to corrode it and this objection may be ignored, particularly as needles should be used only once. A more important disadvantage of iodine is that occasionally patients are hypersensitive to it and develop a dermatitis.

A more complex problem arises from sterilization of the cartridge containing the analgesic solution. Ideally, the entire cartridge should be sterilized by autoclaving, but this method is impractical, as the cartridge bung will blow out. If sterilization of the cartridge is impossible, then certainly the sealing disc which is perforated by the needle when the cartridge is placed in the syringe must be sterilized. This is because organisms present on the sealing disc may be transferred by contact with the needle into the analgesic solution and thus into the tissues. This problem has been partly resolved in various ways.

The simplest answer is to purchase packages of analgesic cartridges which have been sterilized and sealed by the manufacturers, and take care not to contaminate these cartridges during use. The manufacturer has probably employed a method of sterilization which relies on ethylene oxide.

Another method is for the end of the cartridge containing the sealing disc to be dipped in spirit and flamed, but this is not absolutely effective unless it is repeated at least three times.

Antiseptic solutions may also be used to disinfect the cartridge. Correspondence with manufacturers of local analgesics produced the following suggestions: Boots Pure Drug Company recommended complete immersion of the cartridge in 70 per cent alcohol; Astra Chemicals advised immersion of the cartridges in a solution of 0·5 per cent chlorhexidine in 70 per cent ethyl alcohol for 2 minutes; and

Hoechst Pharmaceuticals advised immersion in alcohol or chlorhexidine for about 10 minutes. Astra considered that their method left spores unaffected, but thought it the best and safest for sterilizing cartridges as an immersion time of 2 minutes did not appear long enough for alcohol to penetrate the rubber diaphragm.

A possible disadvantage of these chemical methods, besides that of being ineffective against viruses and spores, was shown in a medicolegal report appearing in 1953 which mentioned the complication of paraplegia, or paralysis of the body below the waist, occurring in two patients following the administration of spinal anaesthetics using analgesic ampoules which had been sterilized by storage in 1 : 40 phenol solution after a temporary immersion in a solution of 1 : 20. The phenol had penetrated the glass to enter the solution and this contamination had caused the paraplegia. Apparently glass is an unusual material in that it may possess cracks which are invisible to the naked eye and permit the penetration of chemical solutions. This complication is less likely to occur with analgesic cartridges which are made of a different type of glass from that used for ampoules. However, a cartridge should always be inspected by the dental surgeon prior to use to check that it is undamaged.

Russell and Lilley (1969) reported on their work regarding contamination of local analgesic cartridges. Three categories were studied: (*a*) as taken from a newly opened carton: (*b*) after 24 hours' exposure to handling in a large teaching clinic; and (*c*) after 5 days' exposure in the same clinic but no handling. The presence of organisms on the diaphragm and metal cap was shown by an impression-plate technique. The terminal centimetre of the cartridge was also sampled by immersion in nutrient broth. The contamination rate for these categories was (*a*) 25 per cent, (*b*) 66 per cent and (*c*) 64 per cent, as determined by immersion technique. Further samples of cartridges treated with 70 per cent alcohol for 5 seconds, 2 minutes and 5 minutes were examined by similar techniques and gave up to 50 per cent positive cultures, while no growth occurred after treatment for 60 minutes.

At the present time there does not appear to be a completely satisfactory answer to the problem of sterilization of the ordinary anal-gesic cartridge. However, by using systems such as the Disposall dental cartridge unit consisting of an analgesic cartridge with hypodermic needle attached as an integral part, the problem of sterilization of the sealing disc is avoided. The ideal answer would be a sterile disposable aspirating syringe already loaded for use and only requiring removal from a protective wrapping just prior to injection. At present, sterile non-aspirating syringes are marketed already filled with drugs including one, Xylocard (Astra), which contains a plain solution of 2 per cent lignocaine for the prevention and treatment of ventricular tachyarrhythmias, so the attainment of this ideal should be possible.

THE MANUFACTURER'S PRECAUTIONS

A description of the production of local analgesic cartridges is given in order to emphasize the care which is taken by the manufacturer in making a sterile cartridge.

The industrial chemist starts with four basic components:

1. The glass cartridge tube.

2. The rubber plunger.

3. Chemicals and distilled pyrogen-free water.

4. The aluminium cap.

Each of these components has to undergo a series of tests and be sterilized before they can all be brought together to form the completed cartridge (*Fig.* 6.4).

1. The glass cartridge tube

First the cartridge tubes have to be tested to eliminate any which may have minute cracks or flaws which would cause them to fracture when under pressure during the administration of an injection. They are also tested chemically, mainly to ensure that no undue alkalinity is present as this would interfere with the stability of the solution. For this reason the glass used should be that described as alkali-free or soda-free.

After they have passed these tests, they are printed with an ink which, ideally, is baked on

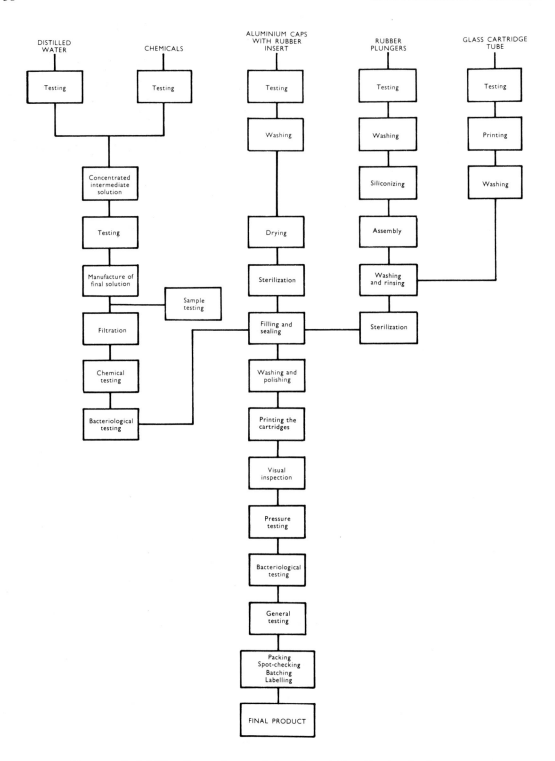

Fig. 6.4. Flow diagram for manufacture of a cartridge of local analgesic.

to the glass to make certain that the record of their contents is permanent. Sometimes pre-printed cartridges are used, these having been produced by the glass manufacturer, or the cartridges may be printed after having been filled as shown in *Fig.* 6.4.

2. Rubber plungers

The plungers are tested and then washed and rinsed. They are then treated with a silicone which lubricates them so that they move smoothly and easily within the glass tube in which they are assembled.

The partially assembled cartridge comprising tube and plunger is now cleaned by 'jetting', a system of high-pressure washing, in a cycle of operations using hot and cold tap-water and distilled water. They are then collected in stainless-steel boxes in which they are steri-lized. Normally, a steam autoclave is used but ethylene oxide sterilization is sometimes employed. The cartridge is now ready to receive its chemicals.

3. Chemicals and water

The chemicals undergo tests for purity before the preparation of the solutions is even started. They are then made up into concentrated solutions using pyrogen-free distilled water as any impurity could affect the chemical stability of the final solution. The final solution is made by diluting the concentrated solutions with distilled water and then mixing them together.

These solutions are:

a. The analgesic.

b. The vasoconstrictor.

c. An antiseptic to maintain the sterility of the solution (*Fig.* 6.5), the exact choice of antiseptic solution depending to a large degree on the stabilizing and buffering agents used in the solution, and also on the types of glass and rubber constituting the cartridge.

d. A stabilizing agent to prevent the break-down of the solution. The stabilization of a solution for injection is a complex matter in-volving many parameters, all of which exhibit degrees of interplay with overlapping effects. Thus the pH is connected with the buffer used,

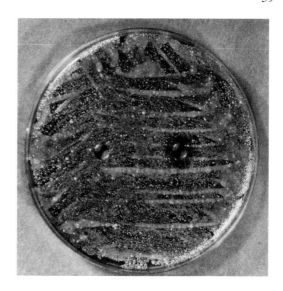

Fig. 6.5. Culture plate showing inhibition of bacterial growth on the right around local analgesic due to its antiseptic, and, on the left, bacterial growth occurring around a control sample of sterile saline.

which in turn is affected by the alkalinity of the glass and rubber components. Similarly, the antiseptic used may be dependent upon the type of rubber from which the plungers are made; chlorocresol, for instance, is very soluble in natural rubber and readily leached from solution by it, whereas hydroxybenzoates are far less likely to be affected.

e. A buffering agent to achieve and maintain the correct pH. This factor has to be be deter-mined very carefully. If the pH is too low then the acidity of the solution will cause pain on injection, whereas if it is too high then in-stability of the analgesic in the solution will result. In determining the kind and quantity of buffer, regard has to be given to the buffering capacity of the tissues, this automatically fixing the upper limit for the quantity of buffer that may be used with the analgesic.

The final solution is now subjected to sample tests and then sterilized by filtration (*Fig.* 6.6). This process uses a filter with an extremely fine mesh of only $0.22\,\mu$m in diameter which will remove bacteria from the solution. The solution is now checked chemically for purity and to verify that the concentrations of the various

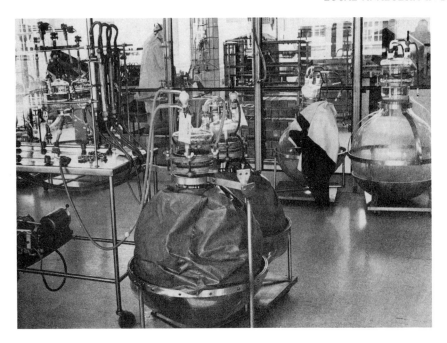

Fig. 6.6. Sterile manufacturing laboratory showing filtration equipment. (*Figs.* 6.6–6.8 reproduced by courtesy of Astra Chemicals Ltd.)

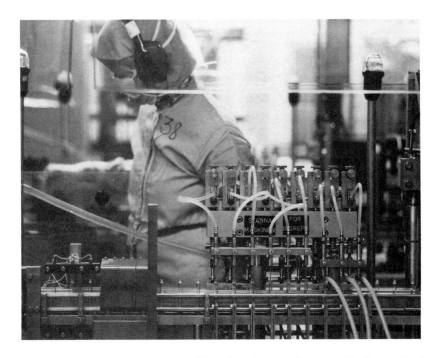

Fig. 6.7. The staff wear gowns, masks, caps, gloves and boots in order to minimize the risk of contaminating the product.

chemicals are correct. Further bacteriological tests ensure that it is sterile and, on passing all these tests, it is ready for insertion in the cartridge.

The loading and sealing of the cartridges are carried out in conditions similar to those considered desirable in an operating theatre. The room is kept as nearly sealed as practicable and the air subjected to a positive pressure by means of an air purifier, thus preventing the ingress of any contaminated air from outside when a door is opened. No staff are allowed to go into this room other than those who actually work there and they are always fully masked, gowned, capped, gloved and booted (*Fig.* 6.7).

4. The aluminium cap

When the solution has been loaded into the cartridge it is sealed by means of an aluminium cap with a rubber insert. Before the caps are used they are subjected to similar checks to the rubber plungers, being washed and sterilized by autoclaving or the use of ethylene oxide.

The final cartridges are washed, polished and then subjected to visual inspection to note any flaws in the quality of the seal or the appearance

of the contents (*Fig.* 6.8). Bacteriological testing is repeated on samples of every batch of the completed cartridges and they are all subjected to a pressure test which is designed to simulate the pressures occurring during an injection. For this purpose an upper limit of 3 kg (6·7 lb) is used, this being the figure suggested by the Australian Commonwealth Bureau of Dental Standards in their official specifications for dental cartridges. The cartridges are now inserted into their final packaging and the boxes labelled and dated. Colour coding is used by most manufacturers for the identification of different solutions, but unfortunately there is no international standardization for this. At this final stage packages are again withdrawn for random checking, including bacteriological culture for sterility.

Nowadays a more compact in-line process may be used in which the components for the cartridge pass through a cleaning machine which includes an ultrasonic bath and then into a drying and sterilization tunnel. From there the components pass directly into an assembling, filling and sealing machine, these units being housed in a sterile room. Also feeding into this machine are two vibrators, one supplying sterilized plungers and the other sterilized caps.

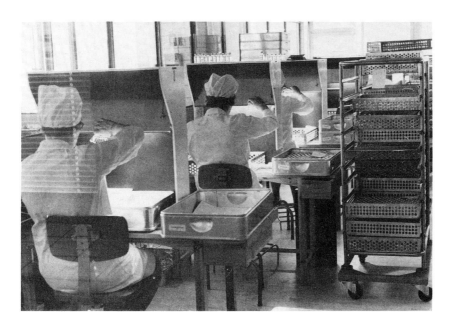

Fig. 6.8. Visual inspection of final products.

REFERENCES AND FURTHER READING

Barnard J. D. W. (1976) Osteomyelitis of the jaws as a sequel to dental local anaesthetic injections. *Br. J. Oral Surg.* **13,** 264.

Blake G. C. and Forman G. H. (1967) Preoperative antiseptic preparation of the oral mucous membrane—a bacteriological assessment. *Br. Dent. J.* **123,** 295.

Kelsey J. C. and Maurer I. M. (1972) *The Use of Chemical Disinfectants in Hospitals.* London, HMSO.

Medicolegal Report (1953) *Br. Med. J.* **2,** 1165.

McLundie A. C., Kennedy G. D. C., Stephen K. W. et al. (1968) Sterilization in general dental practice. *Br. Dent. J.* **124,** 214.

Russell C. and Lilley J. D. (1969) Contamination of local anaesthetic cartridges. IADR (British Division), Abstract No. 73.

Chapter 7

PRECAUTIONS REQUIRED FOR SAFE LOCAL ANALGESIA

The modern local analgesic is extremely safe and contraindications to its use are uncommon; however, these do sometimes occur and thus a careful case history should always be taken to prevent any avoidable complications. When necessary or in doubt the advice of the patient's physician should always be obtained.

CASE HISTORY

The important points to elicit from a patient before commencing any dental treatment will be obtained by asking them their previous medical history (PMH) and previous dental history (PDH).

The PMH should cover:

1. Rheumatic fever, any heart disease and any disorder of blood pressure.
2. Asthma, diabetes and fits.
3. Any other serious illnesses.
4. Previous admissions to hospital, including any operations.
5. Any current medical treatment, together with details of drug therapy, especially steroids, anticoagulants and antidepressants.
6. Drug allergies.

The PDH should include information regarding any ill-effects following the previous administration of local analgesics and pre-medicants, any history of fainting or feeling unwell while having dental treatment, any undue tendency to bruise easily and also details of any excessive postoperative bleeding.

These are the basic inquiries which are used to screen a patient and this chapter will suggest when further information is desirable. Another advantage of a careful case history is that it should provide the operator with a rough assess-ment of the life expectancy of ill and elderly patients, which is very helpful when planning future dental treatment.

AVOIDANCE OF CROSS-INFECTION

More recently the dental profession has become increasingly aware of the need to minimise the risks of cross-infection, especially those associated with hepatitis B, AIDS (Aquired Immune Deficiency Syndrome), and ARC (AIDS-related complex). The PMH may suggest that the patient is a carrier of one of these infections and clinical examination may tend to confirm the diagnosis.

Hepatitis B is discussed on p. 155. AIDS frequently demonstrates cervical lymphadeno-pathy, and a variety of oral manifestations including xerostomia, persistent herpetic ulceration, candidiasis, leukoplakia, and Kaposi's sarcoma, and the patient with ARC has a chronic generalized lymphadenopathy and relapsing fever associated with weight loss and diarrhoea. The high risk groups who may develop AIDS or ARC are promiscuous male homosexuals and bisexuals and their homo-sexual contacts—especially those working as prostitutes, intravenous drug addicts and their sexual partners, and patients who have been unfortunate in receiving contaminated blood transfusions or blood products. The hazards of cross-infection in the dental surgery must be considered from both the need to avoid un-necessary hazards to patients and also the necessity to protect the dental staff. Patients need new sterilized needles and fresh cartridges for local analgesia injections, and staff should have sound knowledge regarding the pre-vention of cross-infection. Vaccination against hepatitis B virus is available to health care personnel, and wearing rubber gloves is a wise precaution when doing surgical work where the patient's blood may come into contact with the operator's hands which usually have minor abrasions and breaches. The management of 'needlestick' injuries is described on p. 155.

CONTRAINDICATIONS TO THE USE OF LOCAL ANALGESIA

General considerations

The administration of a local analgesic implies that the patient's cooperation is required, and for this reason this form of analgesia is not ideal in the very young, very old, severely mentally defective, insane, and also very nervous, excitable and hysterical patients. For the sake of the operator's peace of mind, the treatment of hypercritical patients may be performed more happily if they are given a general anaesthetic. There are some patients who have a very strong objection to knowing what is happening and these people may be unsuitable for the use of local analgesia. With this type of patient, if local analgesia is the only available method which can be employed, then its use may be more successful if the patient is previously premedicated.

Pregnancy

If a woman has a pregnancy which is proceeding normally and her general health is good, there is no reason why she should not have a local analgesic administered. An exception to this rule is that it may be safer to avoid the use of prilocaine, especially with felypressin, for the reasons mentioned in Chapter 4.

However, during pregnancy it is best to restrict routine dental treatment to the middle trimester or 3 months, as it is during this time that complications associated with pregnancy are least likely to occur. The worst time for the pregnant patient to be treated is during the first 3 months at the time of the missed periods.

Occasionally, for example if the patient has toothache, it may be impossible to restrict treatment to this most favourable time and if this situation occurs then it should be kept to the minimum necessary.

Medical conditions

1. Toxaemia

It has been said that in debilitating conditions such as uncontrolled diabetes, nephritis, septicaemia and toxaemia, there is retarded healing. The use of local analgesia causes an additional wound due to the needle track and this may lead to ulceration as the tissues are debilitated. There is also a high risk of secondary infection. This complication can be minimized by giving an antibiotic prophylactically. With fit patients and a sterile technique, the risk of infection causing delayed healing of the needle track is minimal.

2. Haemophilia and other haemorrhagic diatheses

There is an inherent danger when injections are given to patients with severe bleeding diseases. These conditions include haemophilia, Christmas disease, purpura, von Willebrand's disease, and severe liver dysfunction, which often leads to bleeding tendencies. A supraperiosteal injection may cause a haematoma which, although very extensive, is superficial and not usually a danger to life, but an inferior dental block injection may cause deep bleeding into the pterygomandibular region which can track down through the tissue spaces of the neck to cause fatal respiratory obstruction. For this reason the inferior dental, maxillary and posterior superior dental nerve blocks should never be given to these patients and it is safer for injection techniques to be avoided unless used in hospital where continuous surveillance is possible. Here simple extractions are best carried out by means of intraligamentary injections, and conservation performed without local analgesia or under general anaesthesia.

3. Leukaemia

In this blood disorder, especially if it is of the acute variety, two major complications may arise following dental surgery.

Excessive haemorrhage may occur after surgical treatment leading to the sequelae discussed in (2) above. In the leukaemic patient there may be a severe anaemia present so additional blood loss can be serious.

Another complication is the dangerous lowering of resistance which occurs. This may lead to soft-tissue infections and cellulitis which are extremely difficult to control (*Fig.* 7.1).

If a patient with leukaemia requires dental treatment then this should be carried out at a hospital in consultation with the physician caring for the patient.

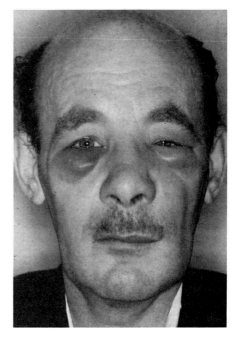

Fig. 7.2. Patient on excessive dose of anticoagulant which led to spontaneous haemorrhage into the soft tissues, epistaxis and haematuria. (Reproduced by courtesy of Professor H. C. Killey and R. C. Bret Day.)

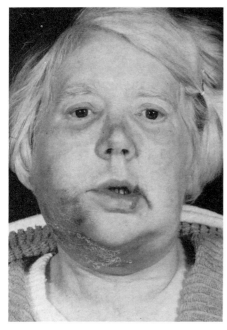

Fig. 7.1. Patient suffering from acute leukaemia who developed a very severe cellulitis with ulceration of the skin following extraction of a lower molar.

4. Anticoagulant therapy

Anticoagulant drugs such as heparin, phenindione (Dindevan, Duncan, Flockhart) and warfarin sodium (Marevan, Duncan, Flockhart) are frequently used in the treatment of coronary artery occlusion and other thrombotic conditions. Patients undergoing this type of therapy usually carry a card describing their treatment and are aware that this therapy may complicate their normal life. The greatest hazard is the risk of excessive haemorrhage if the drug dosage is too high (*Fig.* 7.2). This produces the same type of risk regarding local analgesia as has been described in (2) above.

The dosage level of anticoagulants is usually controlled by periodic estimations of the prothrombin time, and as the dosage needs occasional modification it is prudent to inquire of the patient's physician whether the level is safe for administering injections of local analgesic. Some physicians recommend that their patients stop anticoagulant therapy prior to injections and extractions, whereas others consider that provided the prothrombin time is satisfactory, dental treatment of this type may be performed without altering the dosage of anticoagulants. The numerical value of the prothrombin time at which surgery is free from risks due to anticoagulant therapy will vary depending upon the particular laboratory carrying out the haematological investigation. At present there is no uniformity in the biological materials used for these tests and opinions differ regarding the relative value of these investigations used for assessing anticoagulant therapy. Hence the dental surgeon should confer directly with the haematologist prior to surgical treatment.

In emergency, the risk of excessive haemorrhage may be reduced by giving an antidote to the anticoagulant drug being used; for example, phytomenadione (vitamin K_1) is a direct antagonist to the oral anticoagulants. However, this rapid alteration of the coagulation mechanism of the blood is not without danger as it may institute the complication of 'rebound thrombosis' in which a patient undergoing treatment of a condition such as recurrent venous thrombosis may then be exposed to an increased risk of a further thrombosis.

With any patient undergoing anticoagulant therapy, the advice of his physician should be sought before embarking upon treatment involving the use of local analgesia or any surgical procedure. It is possible when only one or two simple extractions are planned that excessive haemorrhage will be controlled by using antifibrinolytic agents.

Although not directly related to local analgesia, the dental surgeon should not forget other aspects of anticoagulant therapy which are of dental importance. The most notable factor is the modification of the effect of anticoagulants due to the administration of other drugs. For example, many patients receive anticoagulants for treatment of cardiac conditions and because of these same disorders the dental surgeon may choose to prescribe antibiotics. These drugs should not be injected if there is a risk of gross haematoma formation because of the anticoagulant therapy, and if drugs such as ampicillin, tetracycline or penicillin are given orally then theoretically they will interfere with the bacterial flora of the gut so that vitamin K formation is reduced. This deficiency would mean that the anticoagulant action becomes excessive. In practice, this only appears to be significant when antibiotic therapy is used in patients who have gross malnutrition, usually due to some problem of malabsorption.

Other drugs such as the sulphonamides, aspirin, and mixtures containing aspirin, for instance codeine compound tablets, have the same effect. If the dental surgeon wishes to prescribe a drug to relieve pain then the choice should be one such as paracetamol, codeine phosphates or dihydrocodeine bitartrate (DF 118) which does not have any disturbing effect on coagulation.

The ability of drugs to alter the protein binding and metabolism of other drugs has probably been over-emphasized in importance. For example, if warfarin is displaced from its protein binding sites, although there is an initial rise in plasma concentration, warfarin metabolism is increased, so that a new steady state is achieved, and the actual level of increase in plasma concentration is probably very small. However, more important is the synergism of two drugs acting on the same system but at different sites, for example, warfarin decreasing the availability of clotting factors synthesized in the liver, and aspirin decreasing synthesis of thromboxanes in platelets, this substance being important in platelet aggregation.

5. Steroid therapy

Patients on steroid therapy should carry a special record card giving details of their treatment which should be shown by them to their dental surgeon (*Fig. 7.3*).

Patients receiving adrenocortical steroids for conditions such as rheumatoid arthritis, allergic disorders, skin complaints and eye diseases undergo some degree of atrophy of the adrenal

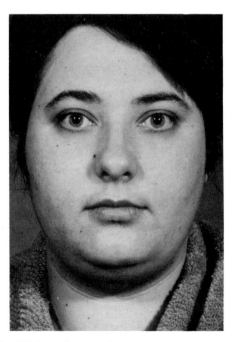

Fig. 7.3. Sometimes a patient who has been on long-term steroid therapy will develop a 'moon face'.

cortex, and because the regeneration of the adrenal tissue is a slow process, the effect of atrophy may still be present even when the steroid therapy was terminated as long ago as 2 years. The atrophy is a more severe process if the steroid dosage has been high and of long duration. Because of the atrophy of the adrenal cortex, the patient's protective mechanism against stress is unable to function properly, and this renders him liable to attacks of faintness, nausea, vomiting and hypotension, which may be fatal. Hence the protection afforded by an increased or additional dosage of adreno-cortical steroid such as hydrocortisone is required. In emergency, if a patient has collapsed and adrenocortical insufficiency is suspected, then the immediate intravenous administration of 200 mg of hydrocortisone sodium succinate may be a life-saving measure.

It is the actual stress which is dangerous to these patients and often the conditions for which local analgesics are administered invoke stress, hence the patient will require the protective cover of additional steroid dosage. When treating these patients their management must be discussed with their physicians because usually extra steroid dosage is indicated prior to the dental treatment and, when this has been completed, the extra steroid dosage is gradually reduced. If problems are anticipated, then the patient should be referred to hospital for emergency treatment which would probably be covered with intravenous steroid therapy.

6. Liver dysfunction

Impairment of liver function may result from infective hepatitis, malaria, cirrhosis or other liver conditions such as secondary carcinomatous deposits. The bleeding tendencies which may occur have been mentioned earlier, but other complications exist, such as infection of the needle wound, which may ensue because the healing processes are poor.

Another danger to the patient arises from the administration of drugs which are detoxicated in the liver because their excretion will be delayed if liver function is impaired. Usually, local analgesia is one of the safest forms of preventing pain in these patients because of the low dosages required. The administration of drugs such as barbiturates, morphine and many of the general anaesthetics should be avoided because of the complications arising from impaired detoxication. Similarly, the Jorgensen technique, mentioned in Chapter 13, which employed pethidine, is undesirable.

The dental surgeon should also consider the safety of his staff and himself. For example, the risks of contracting infections such as viral hepatitis by accidental inoculation via a 'needle-stick' injury in which a sharp instrument such as a syringe needle, probe or root reamer pricks the skin. Protection against some of these infections is available; for instance, there are some specific vaccines against the hepatitis B virus (HBV) and hence it is advisable for a dental practitioner and his nurses to be vaccinated. If a 'needlestick' injury occurs then the injured person may need an injection of immunoglobulin, and if previously vaccinated against HBV, a booster dose of vaccine. If accidental injury occurs then immediate advice regarding management may be sought from a consultant medical microbiologist.

7. Renal disease

Besides the complications due to toxaemia which may arise from nephritis, i.e. uraemia, mentioned in section (1), renal disease can lead to impaired excretion of drugs including local analgesics. This is of particular importance with drugs such as hypnotics and sedatives, of which the barbiturates are a common example.

Uraemia is a type of autointoxication due to the retention of waste products such as urea, uric acid, creatinine and phosphates. The retention of phosphates leads to a fall in the blood calcium level and acidosis.

In patients with liver and renal diseases which are severe enough to contraindicate the use of local analgesia, their prognosis may be so poor that only emergency dental treatment should be considered. For these patients procaine is the ideal analgesic as it is broken down in the plasma.

Local conditions

1. Sepsis

There are some local conditions which preclude the use of an injection technique, the most important of these being sepsis. If a needle is inserted into an acutely inflamed area and an analgesic then administered, the result will be that the solution spreads infection as it diffuses into the tissues. This is a most serious complication, as osteomyelitis or even a fatal cellulitis may ensue. For this reason it is always unwise to administer a local analgesic unless the site of injection can be seen to be healthy. For example, if a posterior superior dental nerve block is to be given, then a mouth mirror should be used to check that the site for injection is uninfected. The reason why the oral mucosa should be dried and painted with an antiseptic prior to injection is that this is another method of reducing the risk of spreading infection. This precaution minimizes the chance of producing what a bacteriologist terms a 'stab culture' in the patient's tissues.

Occasionally, the risk of spreading infection may be reduced by the choice of injection technique. For example, sometimes an injection into an infected area may be avoided by using a regional nerve block instead of injecting the analgesic solution locally.

2. The periostitic tooth

Another condition which contraindicates local analgesia is the treatment of the acutely periostitic tooth. This is because it may be impossible to achieve analgesia of sufficient depth. The reason for this unknown, although various theories have been propounded, which include the following:

a. The pain due to the periostitic tooth produces so many stimuli in the nerve that the local analgesic solution is unable to block the conduction of all these impulses and some of them manage to reach the brain.

b. The pH of the inflammatory products in the region of the tooth is more acidic than usual, thus making the local analgesic solution less effective.

c. Jorgensen (1960) has postulated that as there is a tendency for pain to neutralize the effects of analgesics such as morphine in the central nervous system, there may be a similar explanation for the poor results achieved with local analgesics.

d. Hudson (1960) has mentioned the theory

of a possible spread of inflammation along the myelin sheaths of the nerve which restricts the absorption of the local analgesic.

e. There is usually increased vascularity of the tissues surrounding the periostitic tooth and hence the local analgesic is removed by the bloodstream before it is able to work. Nearer the apex there is vascular stasis so that the analgesic is unable to reach it.

3. Local vascular abnormality

Where there is a local vascular abnormality such as a haemangioma an injection in the region of the lesion should be avoided as the trauma caused by the needle may produce haemorrhage.

CONTRAINDICATIONS DUE TO THE CONSTITUENTS OF THE LOCAL ANALGESIC SOLUTION

Contraindications associated with the analgesic

Epilepsy

Most local analgesics are cerebral stimulants and hence may induce an epileptic attack in a susceptible patient. For this reason epileptics should not be treated under local analgesia unless they are well-stabilized and have taken their usual anticonvulsant drugs, intravenous sedation with diazepam being a useful adjuvant.

Contraindications associated with the vasoconstrictor

1. Cardiovascular disease

It has been stated that adrenaline may precipitate an attack of angina pectoris in patients with myocardial ischaemia but this must be extremely rare. The site of this pain is retrosternal, but it may radiate upwards into the neck and down the arms, especially the ulnar border of the left one, and even into the jaws where it might be misdiagnosed as being of dental origin.

Even in very dilute solutions it is possible for adrenaline to induce cardiac arrhythmias and, very occasionally, ventricular fibrillation and, very rarely, death. Some authorities consider that in hypertensive patients the use of adrenaline should be avoided and that ideally a local analgesic without any vasoconstrictor, such as 2 per cent lignocaine or 4 per cent prilocaine should be employed.

In 1955 a committee of the New York Heart Association produced a report on the use of adrenaline in local analgesia in patients with heart disease and their conclusion was that there is no risk to the patient with heart disease if no more than 0·2 mg of adrenaline is used at a single dental visit. This amount is equivalent to approximately 10 ml of analgesic solution containing 1 : 50 000 adrenaline or 16 ml of solution containing 1 : 80 000 adrenaline. The report did stress that it was desirable for the dental surgeon to contact the patient's physician for information regarding the nature of the cardiac condition and current therapy.

In view of this report, it would seem reasonable to use a local analgesic with a vasoconstrictor for cardiac patients provided that the total volume of solution used is not excessive. The quantities of vasoconstrictor used in local anaesthetic preparations are likely to be insignificant in relation to endogenous release which occurs when stressed. Good analgesia reduces endogenous catecholamine release, and probably the most reliable dental analgesia is generally obtained with 2 per cent lignocaine with 1 : 80 000 adrenaline. Since the report was published, other vasoconstrictors such as felypressin have been discovered, but there is some evidence that that vasoconstrictor actually reduces coronary artery blood flow.

Administration of prophylactic glyceryl trinitrate either sublingually or transdermally may be advised by a physician for those patients with poorly controlled angina and for those who find the prospect of dental treatment particularly anxiety-provoking.

One of the biggest hazards arising from a local anaesthetic solution containing a vasoconstrictor such as adrenaline occurs if the solution is injected intravascularly. Under these conditions, even a small amount of the solution produces a concentration of adrenaline in the bloodstream sufficient to act on the receptors in the aortic arch and carotid sinus. This stimulation produces a sudden rise in blood pressure, and it is the rapidity of this reaction which is particularly disturbing to the patient. This is one of the reasons why local anaesthetic solutions for dental treatment should only be administered with aspirating syringes.

2. Hypertension

This is extremely common, especially in elderly ladies. There are many drugs used to control hypertension, but all act by reducing sympathetic vasomotor activity. Such patients may be treated as normal, but it is advisable to use felypressin as a vasoconstrictor rather than sympathomimetics, although in practice the latter have proved trouble-free.

3. Rheumatic fever

This disease frequently produces the complication of cardiac damage, especially scarring involving the heart valves which develop warty vegetations situated along the areas of contact of the cusps. There are no contraindications to the use of a local analgesic or to the employment of a vasoconstrictor with the analgesic in patients who have had this disease unless cardiovascular damage has occurred, and then intravascular injections must be avoided.

It is important for the dental surgeon to reduce the risk of causing a bacteraemia in a patient who has had rheumatic fever or has a congenital heart defect or a heart murmur. This is because a bacteraemia could lead to organisms settling on the damaged endocardium of the heart valves, thus causing an endocarditis. This complication may be fatal or at best lead to further damage to the already deformed heart valves.

Examples of bacteraemia arising from a dental source include that caused by the movement of mobile teeth which occurs when a patient chews with a dentition which has severe periodontal disease. From this it may be deduced that scaling mobile teeth can cause a bacteraemia. More obviously, any dental treatment which produces a wound, and especially a pumping movement such as occurs during the extraction of a tooth, creates the risk of bacteraemia. Less obviously, exposure of a pulp such as may occur in conservative treatment also produces a similar although probably much lesser risk.

To reduce the chances of bacteraemia occurring a prophylactic bactericidal antibiotic such as penicillin should be administered before treatment so that the blood level of the drug will be raised sufficiently to destroy the organisms. The antibiotic should not be given until shortly before treatment, as otherwise there is time for resistant organisms to develop. In general dental practice a recommended regimen would be to give amoxycillin 3 g orally 1 hour prior to an invasive procedure. Erythromycin is the second-line alternative. High risk groups, such as those with prosthetic valves, require treatment in hospital because they will often need anti-staphylococcal agents such as gentamycin or vancomycin to be given by the intravenous route. It is sometimes a wise precaution to continue the antibiotic cover for a period following treatment if the risk of bacteraemia is likely to persist, for example while a socket is healing, especially if it is known that the attack of rheumatic fever has produced severe cardiac damage. Additionally, the dental surgeon should pay particular attention to local antiseptic procedures in this group of patients such as cleansing the mucosal injection site with a solution of iodine (*see* p. 56).

As a long-term policy, patients who have had rheumatic fever should have their mouths maintained to a very high standard of dental fitness so that the risk of bacteraemia originating from a dental focus is negligible. Some authorities advise that this ideal precludes the retention of non-vital teeth as it is impossible to guarantee that such teeth are sterile. On balance, it would appear that the loss of an equivocal tooth cannot be equated with the potential risk of cardiac damage.

4. Radiation therapy

In patients who have undergone radiation therapy by deep X-rays, radium needles or radon seeds, special care will be required if the jaws have been irradiated and surgery is to be performed. The effect of irradiation on bone is to reduce its blood supply due to fibrosis of the bone marrow. Because healing of bone depends upon a good blood supply, it is prudent to avoid the use of anything such as a local analgesic solution containing a vasoconstrictor which tends to reduce that blood supply. This may

sound a drastic suggestion, but irradiated bone is a treacherous tissue which has a poor resistance and infection can lead to osteoradionecrosis with massive sequestration.

The problems concerning the healing of irradiated bone should become fewer now that new techniques involving supervoltage machines, teleradium—which is the use of a large amount of radium in a special unit—and, more recently, radioactive elements such as cobalt-60 are employed. In addition to these new methods, the serious complications arising from haphazard irradiation of bone are now understood and specialist physicists are employed in radiotherapy departments to calculate accurately the dosage and direction of the beam. With these precautions it is possible to localize the radiation to just the tumour site and successfully treat a tumour without adversely affecting any bone which may be intervening between the source of radiation and the lesion. Thus the capacity of the bone to respond to infection with a normal inflammatory reaction is not impaired. Another improvement which has occurred is that most radiotherapists will refer their patients to a dental surgeon for the elimination of oral sepsis prior to treatment if the jaw bones are likely to be irradiated. The dental surgeon should be very critical of any teeth remaining in the patient's mouth, and if there is any doubt at all then a clearance should be performed. An irradiated mouth frequently becomes a dry mouth due to the effects of radiation on the salivary glands and under these conditions the caries rate is increased and the loss of teeth accelerated.

5. Hyperthyroidism

These patients may be extremely nervous and emotional and therefore unable to provide the cooperation which is necessary when undergoing treatment under local analgesia.

If this method is employed then adrenaline and other sympathomimetic vasoconstrictors should not be administered as the patient may have an increased sensitivity to them and their use may precipitate a toxic crisis. Even a very small amount of adrenaline may make the patient feel unwell with tachycardia, faintness and chest pain. Felypressin is the vasoconstrictor of choice.

A patient with active thyrotoxicosis should be premedicated if treatment under local analgesia is necessary, but there are no special problems if the thyrotoxicosis has been treated. Because liver function is sometimes impaired in hyperthyroidism, the dental surgeon should avoid administering drugs such as barbiturates which are detoxicated in the liver.

6. Diabetes mellitus

This is a common metabolic disease in which the blood-sugar level sometimes becomes raised to such a degree that sugar is excreted in the urine. Fortunately, it is a disorder which may be successfully treated by diet, insulin and drugs such as the sulphonylureas which lower the blood-sugar level. In general, those with mild diabetes are controlled by diet alone, more severe diabetics take oral hypoglycaemic drugs, and the most severe ones take insulin. There are no complete contraindications to the use of local analgesia with or without a vasoconstrictor on the well-controlled diabetic patient.

Although adrenaline and, to a lesser extent, noradrenaline raise the blood-sugar level by stimulating the breakdown of liver glycogen into glucose, there is such a weak concentration of these vasoconstrictors present in local analgesic solutions that their glycogenolytic action may be safely ignored.

In dental and oral surgery there are three important considerations when treating diabetics. First, do not treat them unless they are well-stabilized or under the care of a physician who has agreed to the dental treatment which is contemplated; secondly, remember that they are more prone to infection and therefore an antibiotic cover is desirable for all surgical treatment; and thirdly, operations on the teeth and oral cavity may make it difficult for diabetic patients to eat and thus care should be taken to ensure that they are able to maintain their correct carbohydrate intake. This aspect is most important and therefore the diabetic should be advised not to starve prior to having treatment under local analgesia and if, following this, the mouth is sore, then the carbohydrate intake should be maintained in the form of a fluid diet. The ideal time for treatment under local analgesia would be shortly after the patient has had his antidiabetic treatment.

Interaction between drugs

1. Tricyclic antidepressants

These drugs are very widely used for treating depression and sometimes for treating nocturnal enuresis in children.

Those in use include the following:

Approved Name	Proprietary Name
Amitriptyline	Domical (Berk)
	Lentizol (Parke, Davis)
	Limbitrol (Roche)
	Tryptizol (Merck Sharp & Dohme)
Amitriptyline with perphenazine	Triptafen-DA (Allen & Hanburys)
Butriptyline hydrochloride	Evadyne (Ayerst)
Clomipramine	Anafranil (Geigy)
Desipramine hydrochloride	Pertofran (Geigy)
Dothiepin	Prothiaden (Boots)
Doxepin hydrochloride	Sinequan (Pfizer)
Imipramine hydrochloride	Praminil (DDSA Pharmaceuticals)
	Tofranil (Geigy)
Iprindole	Prondol (Wyeth)
Nortriptyline	Aventyl (Lilly)
	Allegron (Dista)
Nortriptyline hydrochloride with fluphenazine	Motival (Squibb)
Protriptyline hydrochloride	Concordin (Merck Sharp & Dohme)
Trimipramine acid maleate	Surmontil (May & Baker)

The tricyclic antidepressants interact with noradrenaline so that its systemic effects are increased by amounts reported as varying from fourfold to about ninefold, and with adrenaline to a lesser extent. As noradrenaline in these circumstances causes a marked rise in blood pressure, and adrenaline increases the heart rate and may alter its rhythm, these side-effects are potentially dangerous and therefore local anaesthetic solutions containing noradrenaline or adrenaline should not be used on patients taking tricyclic drugs. Instead, it would be safe either to use a solution containing a non-amine vasoconstrictor such as felypressin, which is available with the local analgesic prilocaine or, for shorter periods of treatment, to use an analgesic solution without a vasoconstrictor such as plain prilocaine or mepivacaine.

2. Tetracyclic antidepressants

These constitute a newer group of antidepressant drugs which produce the same type of interaction with the sympathomimetic amines adrenaline and noradrenaline as do the tricyclics. They are thought to have the advantage that they do not interfere with uptake-1, the presynaptic system by which catecholamine neurotransmitters are removed, and therefore they are theoretically safer than tricyclics.

Tetracyclic antidepressants in use include:

Approved Name	Proprietary Name
Maprotiline hydrochloride	Ludiomil (Ciba)
Mianserin hydrochloride	Bolvidon (Organon) Norval (Bencard)

3. Monoamine oxidase inhibitors (MAOIs)

These antidepressant drugs are used much less frequently now because of hazardous dietary and drug interactions, the tricyclic antidepressants being the drugs of choice for treating depressive illness with the MAOIs being prescribed when tricyclics are unsuccessful.

Those in use include the following:

Approved Name	Proprietary Name
Iproniazid	Marsilid (Roche)
Isocarboxazid	Marplan (Roche)
Pargyline (USNF)	Eutonyl (Abbott)
Phenelzine	Nardil (Warner)
Tranylcypromine	Parnate (Smith Kline & French)
Tranylcypromine and trifluoperazine	Parstelin (Smith Kline & French)

Often patients are not aware of the identity of drugs which they have been prescribed, but the dental surgeon may get a clue from the fact that patients receiving monoamine oxidase inhibitors should have been warned about their diet. Cheese is a potentially dangerous food for these patients as the monoamine oxidases in the alimentary tract and liver are inhibited and this permits the absorption of tyramine from ingested cheese. A sudden rise in blood pressure may result because of the release of noradrenaline from adrenergic nerves due to the circulating tyramine. The hypertensive episode may cause severe headache or even acute heart failure or intracranial haemorrhage. Other foods such as broad beans, which contain dopa, and yeast extracts such as Marmite or Bovril may cause the same adverse effects.

Dangerous reactions may occur when sympathomimetic drugs are administered, and therefore from the dental aspect it was originally thought that adrenaline and noradrenaline should not be used as vasoconstrictors with these patients. However, it has been stated in the British Dental Formulary, 1968, that the minute amounts used in local analgesic solutions are of no danger to such patients. Some published reports were sceptical about the inherent dangers of monoamine oxidase inhibitors, and it is probable that the potentiation of adrenaline or noradrenaline does not occur to a great extent as these are also broken down by catechol-o-methyltransferase.

Analgesic mixtures and sprays, used for constricting the nasal mucosa or dilating the bronchi, and which contain amphetamine, dextro-amphetamine, methylamphetamine or ephedrine should be avoided, and there is also danger in administering morphine, pethidine and barbiturates because their actions may be potentiated by monoamine oxidase inhibitors. Thus these drugs must always be avoided and premedication with barbiturates and the Jorgensen technique are contraindicated. These complications may occur up to 3 weeks after the monoamine oxidase inhibitor therapy has been discontinued as these drugs are only slowly excreted.

The complication of excessive hypertension which occurs with sympathomimetics may be treated by injecting an adrenergic blocking drug such as phentolamine or chlorpromazine to block the peripheral nerve receptors. The usual dose of phentolamine is 5–10 mg intravenously, but more may be needed if the blood pressure remains raised. The severe hypotension which results from the administration of pethidine or morphine may be treated with hydrocortisone hemisuccinate 100 mg intravenously. With either of these complications the patient should be transferred to hospital for continued observation.

4. Sulphonamides

These chemotherapeutic drugs and also some of the sulphonamide derivatives which are used orally in the treatment of diabetes mellitus are derivatives of *para*-aminobenzoic acid. In a similar way local analgesics such as procaine and amethocaine have the same chemical derivation from the *para*-aminobenzoic acid ring, and following an injection of procaine, hydrolysis occurs back to *para*-aminobenzoic acid due to the enzyme procaine esterase which is present in the liver and circulating blood. When a local analgesic of this type is used on a patient receiving sulphonamides, antagonism occurs between the drugs so that theoretically both become ineffective, although this has not been substantiated in practice. Other local analgesics such as lignocaine and prilocaine have a different chemical derivation and are the drugs of choice for patients on sulphonamides. If a patient has a hypersensitivity to these drugs, then it is probably due to the *para*-aminobenzoic acid ring and therefore it is necessary to avoid the use of local analgesics with the same basic chemical structure as the patient could also be hypersensitive to these.

5. General anaesthetics

Occasionally during an operation under general anaesthesia the surgeon will wish to secure a bloodless field by infiltrating into the tissues a local analgesic solution containing a vasoconstrictor. Some general anaesthetic agents such as cyclopropane, halothane and trichloroethylene sensitize the heart so that cardiac arrhythmia—which may lead to cardiac arrest—can occur if adrenaline or possibly noradrenaline is administered. To avoid complications of this sort the surgeon should always check with the anaesthetist before injecting a local analgesic solution. Felypressin may be used instead of adrenaline but is not as effective in producing vasoconstriction.

6. Cocaine and sympathomimetic drugs

One of the side-effects of cocaine is to potentiate the action of adrenaline and thus produce a sympathomimetic response, probably by combining with the enzyme amine oxidase to prevent it from oxidizing adrenaline and noradrenaline. Thus, if cocaine is absorbed from the oral or nasal mucosa of a patient taking a sympathomimetic such as amphetamine, then complications in the form of cardiac arrhythmias or convulsions may occur.

Similarly, ephedrine-containing cold cures which may be purchased over the counter without prescription are a more commonly encountered problem than amphetamines, mainly because patients do not regard them as drugs which they should declare. Ephedrine has indirect sympathomimetic actions, and will therefore potentiate the effect of cocaine which is still used as a topical anaesthetic in certain special circumstances.

REFERENCES AND FURTHER READING

Boakes A. J., Laurence D. R., Teoh P. C. et al. (1973) Interactions between sympathomimetic amines and antidepressant agents in man. *Br. Med. J.* **1,** 311.

Dinsdale R. C. W. (1985) Viral hepatitis, AIDS and dental treatment. London: *The British Dental Journal.*

Hudson M. W. P. (1960) *Digest Report of the Meeting of the Society for the Advancement of Anaesthesia in Dentistry,* 1 December, 1960.

Jorgensen N. B. (1960) *Digest Report of the Society for the Advancement of Anaesthesia in Dentistry,* 1 December, 1960.

McIver A. K. (1967) Drug interactions. *Pharm. J.* **199,** 205.

Report of the Special Committee of the New York Heart Association (1955) *J. Am. Dent. Assoc.* **50,** 108.

Chapter 8

SURFACE ANALGESIA

The topical application of analgesics has many uses, ranging from a mild, generalized desensitization of the oral cavity prior to the taking of impressions, to the localized numbing of the mucous membrane before incising an abscess.

The main methods of application are:

  a. In mouthwashes.
  b. In lozenges.
  c. Topical application of pastes and solutions.
  d. By sprays.
  e. By jet injector.
  f. By refrigeration.

There is some overlap between groups (*a*) and (*c*), as sometimes the same product may be used as a mouthwash or by topical application.

It must be remembered that surface analgesics are extremely rapidly absorbed systemically and thus should be used with care, their absorption being almost equivalent to intravascular administration. This rapid absorption has led to toxic side-effects, particularly when used in conjunction with injections of local anaesthetic solutions, and hence topical analgesics must be used with care. Several fatalities have been reported by Adriani and Campbell (1956) and Adriani and Dalili (1971), but these have been when topical analgesics were used in large dosages prior to procedures such as bronchoscopy. In all these cases the total dosage of the surface analgesic grossly exceeded the accepted safe dose.

MOUTHWASHES AND LOZENGES

The commonest use of these is for a patient who has a 'sensitive palate' and experiences difficulty in tolerating dental treatment of any type, particularly having impressions taken. Another use is for relieving pain in cases of severe aphthous and other forms of ulceration of the oral mucosa. If used immediately prior to a meal, they enable a patient to eat with some degree of comfort, although care should be taken to avoid making the mouth so numb that it is traumatized during mastication.

An example of a mouthwash used to alleviate pain is a 4 per cent solution of lignocaine hydrochloride which can be rinsed around the mouth and then expelled. For topical use the maximum dose of 4 per cent lignocaine hydrochloride is 5 ml if the solution does not contain a vasoconstrictor and up to 12·5 ml if it does.

Analgesic lozenges commonly used are benzocaine (DPF) which each contain benzocaine 10 mg, and compound benzocaine (BPC, BNF) which each contain benzocaine 100 mg and menthol 3 mg. It is customary to dispense 25 of the benzocaine lozenges or 10 of the compound benzocaine lozenges unless otherwise stated. Dequacaine (Farley) lozenges each contain benzocaine 10 mg and dequalinium chloride 250 μg, the latter being sometimes prescribed on its own for treating mild fungal infections. The maximum daily dosage is eight lozenges. Benzocaine is comparatively non-irritant and non-toxic, the usual fatal dose being about 12 g, although death has been reported with smaller amounts. It is important not to confuse benzocaine lozenges with compound benzocaine lozenges which each contain 10 times as much benzocaine. A lozenge containing 200 mg of lignocaine is available, but for most dental purposes a half to a quarter of this dosage is sufficient. Lignocaine is also available in an oral gel, Oral-B, which contains lignocaine 0·6 per cent, cetylpyridinium chloride 0·02 per cent, cineole 0·1 per cent and menthol 0·06 per cent. It may be applied to painful oral lesions at 3-hourly intervals when required.

PASTES AND SOLUTIONS

Method of use
These are applied according to their consistency. Usually the solutions are rinsed around the mouth and allowed to bathe a particular region of the oral mucosa or are painted on with an applicator such as a pledget of cotton-wool, whereas the pastes are actively massaged on to the mucosa after previously drying it.

A slightly different mode of administration is necessary when the antihistamine diphenhydramine is used. This is employed as an analgesic mouthwash by mixing a 50-mg capsule of it in a teaspoonful of water and holding this in the mouth for 3 minutes. The solution is then swallowed and absorbed so that its sedative action is obtained. This drug is used for the relief of symptoms caused by various forms of painful oral ulceration.

Indications
The main use of this group of analgesics is *topical application prior to an injection* and, with their aid and a careful technique, most infiltration injections may be given quite painlessly.

Other uses of pastes and solutions are listed below:

1. For *minor surgical procedures,* such as the extraction of very loose deciduous teeth and removal of small superficial sequestrae. It should be remembered that in these cases the administration of an injection such as the inferior dental nerve block may cause more discomfort than the treatment, even without analgesia.

2. For the *incision of an abscess.* In these cases it may be impossible to use an injection technique for fear of spreading the infection into deeper tissues. For the incision, a sharp scalpel should always be used to minimize pain arising from the deeper tissues due to excessive pressure.

3. For *deep scaling.* This can be quite a painful procedure and the use of topical analgesia eases the patient's discomfort and thus enables the operation to be carried out more thoroughly. The gingival margins should be isolated, dried and the paste massaged well down into the pockets.

Contents
The drugs commonly used for achieving surface analgesia are cinchocaine, amethocaine, benzocaine and lignocaine, and two or more of these are generally combined.

Typical pastes contain 5 per cent lignocaine and 2 per cent amethocaine in a water-miscible base, or 5 per cent lignocaine with the addition of 0·015 per cent hyaluronidase, which is an enzyme aiding the passage of the analgesic through the surface mucosa (*see* p. 30). A less effective paste is compound benzocaine ointment, BPC, which contains 10 per cent of benzocaine in equal parts of hamamelis and zinc ointment.

Analgesic solutions include 0·5–2 per cent amethocaine hydrochloride, 0·5–2 per cent cinchocaine hydrochloride, 5–10 per cent cocaine hydrochloride and 4 per cent lignocaine hydrochloride.

The time taken for the onset of surface analgesia is at least 2 minutes; however, it should be remembered that the speed of onset and depth of analgesia achieved depend entirely on the permeability of the mucosa to which it is applied, and this is directly related to the degree of keratinization present. Thus it is most effective at the site of a buccal infiltration, less effective in the palate and would be quite useless on the palm of the hand.

It is wise to avoid undue contact with the surface analgesics as it is relatively common for an operator to develop a sensitivity to some of these drugs. Amethocaine is a frequent offender, but fortunately lignocaine rarely causes this trouble.

EUTECTIC CREAMS

Dr Hans Evers and his colleagues have introduced a new type of surface anaesthetic cream (EMLA) based on the eutectic mixture of lignocaine and prilocaine. At present two strengths,

2·5 per cent and 5 per cent, have been used by applying it to the skin for 1 hour after which the area is found to be analgesic to testing by pinprick. This has enabled intravenous cannulas to be inserted painlessly which indicates that EMLA will be useful for applying to skin sites prior to venepuncture, possibly in the form of an adhesive medicated dressing, and may be particularly valuable for children and nervous patients. In the past, analgesia of the skin has been difficult to obtain with a surface application due to the thickness of the keratinized dermis restricting absorption of anaesthetic drugs. There have been no reports of skin reactions from repeated applications, and plasma concentrations of lignocaine and prilocaine have remained low.

ANALGESIC SPRAYS

These are usually supplied in aerosol form and have two principal uses:

1. *Prior to deep scaling.*
2. *For spraying on to the palate before taking an impression.* However, care must be exercised in using it for this purpose because if the spray is applied for too long or while the patient is inhaling, then it may pass down into the larynx and cause distress. The spray should not be applied for longer than 1 second.

Lignocaine is marketed as a spray and one squirt or spray contains about 10 mg, 20 squirts being the maximum recommended dose on a mucous membrane.

JET INJECTORS

These may be used for two purposes:

1. *For obtaining surface analgesia.*
2. *For producing deeper penetration of the tissues* so that they may be used in place of the conventional infiltration injection.

In both cases the basic method is the 'firing' of analgesic solution at the surface mucosa or skin by means of compressed gas so that a fine jet of solution is able to penetrate the tissues (*Figs.* 8.1, 8.2). In cases where surface analgesia is required the force needs to be just sufficient for the solution to raise a small 'bleb' on the surface tissues, analgesia occurring within a few seconds. The amount of solution and the force applied to it are carefully metered by the gun, 0·04 ml in the case of the Panjet being all that is required to produce an area of analgesia of 5 mm diameter, which gradually spreads to about 1 cm diameter within a few minutes. The Mizzy Syrijet can inject up to 0·2 ml of solution into the tissues at one time and thus the area of analgesia is increased proportionally. This is of particular value prior to an infiltration injection, especially on the palatal mucosa where tissue is firmly bound to the underlying bone by fibrous septa.

The jet injector is also of use in obtaining a localized area of analgesia for techniques such as taking an impression for bridgework, thus obviating the need for a hypodermic or hypomucosal injection. To reach a tooth the solution has to pass into deeper tissues and larger quantities of analgesic solution are required,

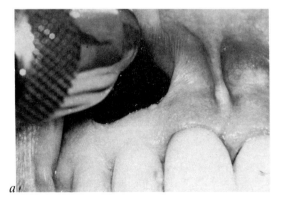
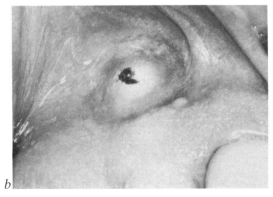

a   *b*

Fig. 8.1. *a,* Jet injector being used in the labial sulcus with the rubber cone in contact with the mucous membrane. *b,* The same site immediately after injection showing the weal, blanching and a spot of blood at the puncture wound. (*Figs.* 8.1, 8.2 reproduced from Whitehead F. I. H. and Young I. (1968) *Br. Dent. J.* **125,** 437.)

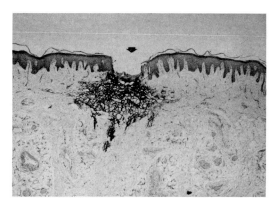

Fig. 8.2. Section of human mucosa showing the puncture wound and the limited penetration of the jet-injected solution.

these being given by multiple shots. Any local analgesic solution suitable for injection may be used in a jet injector.

REFRIGERATION

The principle of this method is the lowering of the temperature of the tissues to achieve analgesia. This is easily understood if one thinks of the peculiar lack of sensation of the fingers if they become very cold—indeed, they are 'numb with the cold'.

The method commonly employed to achieve chilling of the tissues is by spraying on a volatile material such as ethyl chloride. As this evaporates, it removes heat from the tissues due to its

latent heat of evaporation and thus chills them. Analgesia is achieved by this method when a white frost appears on the surface of the tissues. If this is being used at the back of the mouth, then a gauze pack should be placed posterior to the site of application to discourage the inhalation of this drug which is also a general anaesthetic. Care must be taken to avoid spraying so much ethyl chloride that the patient loses consciousness.

The main uses of this method are for the incision of an acute abscess where an injection technique is precluded, or for removing a very loose tooth.

The main disadvantages are:

1. Difficulty of application, especially in the back of the mouth.
2. The inhalation by the patient of the ethyl chloride fumes.
3. The discomfort caused if the chilling ethyl chloride touches sensitive teeth.
4. The extremely short duration of analgesia.

REFERENCES AND FURTHER READING

Adriani J. and Campbell D. (1956) Fatalities following topical application of local anaesthetics to mucous membranes. *JAMA* **162,** 1527.

Adriani J. and Dalili H. (1971) Penetration of local anaesthetics through epithelial barriers. *Anaesth. Analg. (Cleve.)* **50,** 834.

Evers H., Von Dardel O., Juhlin L. et al. (1985) Dermal effects of compositions based on the eutectic mixture of lignocaine and prilocaine (EMLA). Studies in volunteers. *Br. J. Anaesth.* **57,** 997.

Chapter 9

ANATOMY IN RELATION TO LOCAL ANALGESIA

The only nerve with which the dental surgeon is concerned when administering a local analgesic is the trigeminal, which is the largest of the cranial nerves (*Fig.* 9.1.). This has a big sensory and a small motor root. It supplies the mandible, maxilla and associated structures, and also most of the skin of the face. The motor branch supplies all the muscles of mastication but not the buccinator, which is considered to be a muscle of facial expression, being innervated by the facial nerve.

Both the sensory and motor nuclei lie fairly

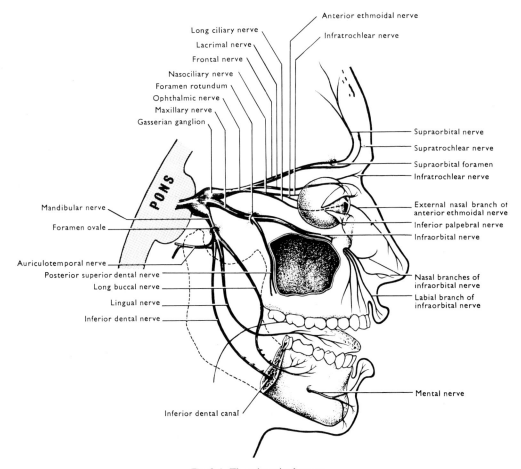

Fig. 9.1. The trigeminal nerve.

near to the middle of the pons. The fibres from the motor root pass forwards and laterally in the posterior cranial fossa and run immediately below the Gasserian ganglion to reach the foramen ovale through which they pass before joining the mandibular division.

From the nucleus in the pons the sensory root runs forwards and laterally to the middle cranial fossa. Here it reaches a large ganglion, the Gasserian, which is located at the apex of the petrous portion of the temporal bone and lies in the cave of Meckel, which is a prolongation of the dura mater from the posterior cranial fossa. From this ganglion the three divisions of the trigeminal nerve arise: the ophthalmic from the anterior part, the maxillary from the middle and the mandibular from the posterior part.

THE OPHTHALMIC OR FIRST DIVISION OF THE TRIGEMINAL NERVE

This nerve, which is entirely sensory, is of little interest to the dental surgeon. It divides into three main branches which pass into the orbit through the superior orbital fissure. These are:

1. The *lacrimal nerve*. This is the smallest of the branches. It supplies the gland of the same name, the fibres being parasympathetic in nature and reaching the lacrimal nerve via the sphenopalatine ganglion. It also supplies part of the upper eyelid and the corresponding part of the conjunctiva.

2. The *frontal nerve*. This supplies the forehead and the scalp as far back as the vertex. It also supplies the skin at the root of the nose, the skin and conjunctiva of the upper eyelid, and the mucosal lining of the frontal sinus.

3. The *nasociliary nerve*. This supplies the cornea and sclera of the eye, the upper and anterior part of the nasal septum, and the lateral wall of the nose.

THE MAXILLARY OR SECOND DIVISION OF THE TRIGEMINAL NERVE

This division is entirely sensory (*Fig.* 9.2). It supplies the whole of the maxilla including the teeth and their gingivae, the maxillary sinus, and the mucous membranes of the hard and soft palates, the nasal cavity and the nasopharynx. In addition, it innervates the skin of the upper lip, the upper part of the cheek, the lower eyelid, and the adjacent part of the nose, the skin over the anterior part of the temporal region, and that overlying the zygomatic bone.

From the Gasserian ganglion the maxillary nerve runs forward in the lateral wall of the cavernous sinus and passes through the foramen

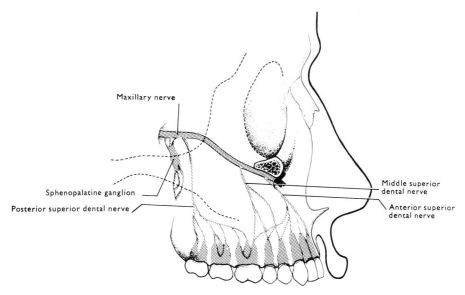

Fig. 9.2. The maxillary nerve.

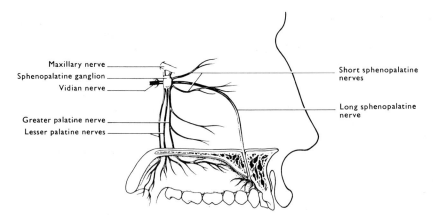

Fig. 9.3. Branches of the maxillary nerve passing through the sphenopalatine ganglion.

rotundum to reach the pterygopalatine fossa. From the maxillary nerve at this point is suspended the sphenopalatine ganglion which is part of the parasympathetic system (*Fig.* 9.3). *Through the sphenopalatine ganglion pass the following main branches:*

1. To the *orbit*.

2. The *short sphenopalatine nerves* reach the nose via the sphenopalatine foramen. They supply the upper and posterior part of the lateral wall of the nose.

3. The *long sphenopalatine (nasopalatine) nerve* (*Fig.* 9.3) passes along the septum, which it supplies, to the floor of the nasal cavity, and then through the incisive canal to emerge at the incisive fossa on to the palate. It supplies the mucoperiosteum, gingivae and alveolar process of the anterior part of the palate (*Fig.* 9.4).

4. The *greater palatine nerve* gains the palate by passing through the greater palatine foramen

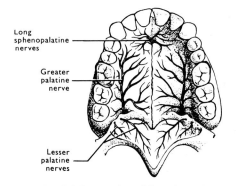

Fig. 9.4. Innervation of the palate.

which is situated medially to the second or third molar. It supplies the mucoperiosteum and gingivae of the hard palate from the canine posteriorly and rarely may supply the palatal roots of the maxillary first and second molars. This explains why there are occasions when maxillary molars remain sensitive after buccal infiltration injections have been given and analgesia is not obtained until additional palatal infiltrations have been administered.

5. The *lesser palatine nerves* traverse the lesser palatine foramina of the hard palate to innervate the mucosa of the soft palate and the uvula. The palatine nerves together supply the whole of the sensory innervation to the mucosa, covering the hard and soft palates, and also propagate secretory and taste fibres to this region.

6. A small *pharyngeal branch* passes from the ganglion to reach the nasopharynx.

The maxillary nerve, after giving off stout branches to the sphenopalatine ganglion, immediately gives off two further branches:

a. The *zygomatic nerve* which passes through the inferior orbital fissure where it divides into a temporal branch supplying the skin of the temporal region and a facial branch supplying the skin over the zygomatic bone. Secretory fibres pass from the sphenopalatine ganglion with the zygomatic nerve, and then leave it to reach the lacrimal gland. These fibres do not originate from the trigeminal nerve but merely accompany the sensory zygomatic nerve fibres.

b. The *posterior superior dental nerve* or

nerves are variable in number and pass downwards on the posterior aspect of the maxilla and enter it approximately 1 cm above and behind the third molar. However, before doing so, they give off gingival branches to supply the buccal gingivae of the upper molars. After entering bone they divide into branches which supply all the innervation for the upper molars, except sometimes the mesiobuccal root of the first molar which may be supplied by the *middle superior dental nerve*. This nerve, which is present in only approximately 50 per cent of patients, combines with the anterior and posterior superior dental nerves to form a plexus which is sometimes termed the 'outer nerve loop'.

The maxillary nerve now traverses the inferior orbital fissure to reach the orbit where it lies in the infraorbital groove outside the orbital periosteum and thus, strictly speaking, outside the orbit. Here it becomes known as the infraorbital nerve and then passes into the infraorbital canal. It is here that it gives off the middle superior dental nerve which, when present, runs down in the lateral wall of the maxillary sinus, to which it gives off twigs. It supplies both premolars and also the mesiobuccal root of the first molar. When absent, the supply to the premolars is taken over by the fibres of the anterior superior dental nerve.

The *anterior superior dental nerve* is given off approximately 5 mm before the external end of the infraorbital canal and supplies the incisor and canine teeth and also the anterior part of the maxillary sinus and nose. The infraorbital nerve escapes from the front of the maxilla through the infraorbital foramen. At this point an infraorbital nerve block is readily administered as the fluid will diffuse back through the canal to reach the anterior superior dental nerve. The infraorbital nerve now divides into its terminal branches, which are:

i. *Palpebral*, passing to the skin of the lower eyelid and associated conjunctiva.
ii. *Nasal* branches to the skin of the side of the nose.
iii. *Labial* branches to the skin and mucous membrane of the upper lip, the labial gingivae and the vestibule of the nose.

THE MANDIBULAR OR THIRD DIVISION OF THE TRIGEMINAL NERVE

This division of the trigeminal nerve is both sensory and motor (*Fig.* 9.5), supplying all the muscles of mastication. The sensory part innervates the whole of the lower jaw including the teeth and their associated gingivae, the skin

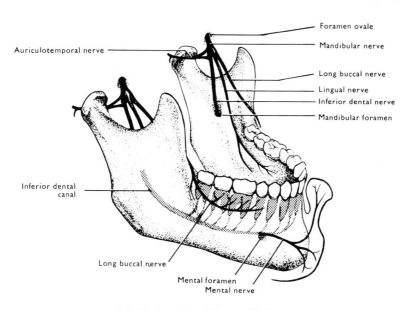

Fig. 9.5. The branches of the mandibular nerve.

overlying the chin, the skin and mucous membrane of the lower lip and part of the cheek, and the anterior two-thirds of the tongue, except for the circumvallate papillae.

The sensory part of the nerve leaves the Gasserian ganglion at its posterolateral border and passes out of the skull through the foramen ovale. After doing so it is joined by the smaller motor root which runs below the ganglion. As the mandibular nerve leaves the skull it lies on the tensor palati muscle and is covered by the lateral pterygoid muscle. Almost as soon as it has passed through the foramen a small motor branch is given off to supply the medial pterygoid. This nerve proceeds to the otic ganglion, which it surrounds, and then supplies the tensor palati and tensor tympani. After this the mandibular nerve divides into a large posterior and a smaller anterior division.

The anterior division of the mandibular nerve

This is mainly motor but has a sensory component. It divides early in its course to supply motor fibres to:

 a. The lateral pterygoid.
 b. The masseter.
 c. The temporalis via two branches.

Its only sensory branch is the *long buccal nerve.* This passes down between the two heads of the lateral pterygoid to reach the anterior border of the masseter, behind and at a similar occlusal level to the third molar with the mouth closed. However, when the mouth is open, the nerve moves below the level of the upper third molar and this is one site where it can be conveniently 'blocked'.

It now divides, some fibres piercing the buccinator to supply the buccal gingivae of the posterior region and also part of the mucous membrane of the oral aspect of the cheek, and other fibres continuing forwards to supply the skin of the cheek.

Posterior division of the mandibular nerve

This is mainly sensory and passes downwards medial to the lateral pterygoid, where it gives off three branches, the lingual, inferior dental and auriculotemporal nerves.

The lingual nerve

This passes down deep to the lateral pterygoid and on the surface of the medial pterygoid. When it reaches the lower border of the lateral pterygoid it is anterior to the inferior dental nerve. Here it is joined by the chorda tympani which conveys the sense of taste from the anterior two-thirds of the tongue. This nerve originates from the facial nerve from which it is given off in the temporal bone. The lingual nerve then runs downwards and forwards, taking up a position just deep to the mucous membrane on the inner aspect of the third molar a little above the mylohyoid line. Its position here is of considerable surgical importance as it may be easily damaged when removing lingual bone prior to elevating out a third molar.

The lingual nerve continues downwards and forwards and divides into branches supplying the mucous membrane of the floor of the mouth, the gingivae on the lingual aspects of the teeth and the anterior two-thirds of the tongue, except for the circumvallate papillae.

The inferior dental nerve

This nerve passes down deep to the lateral pterygoid, where it is separated from the medial pterygoid by the sphenomandibular ligament, to reach the mandibular foramen, at which site it may be 'blocked'. However, Sicher and DuBrul (1975) record that one or more branches of the inferior dental nerve are occasionally given off before the foramen is reached and enter the bone through auxiliary foramina in front of and above the mandibular foramen. These probably supply the third molar and it is this aberrant nerve supply which occasionally causes failure of an inferior dental nerve block.

Before entering the foramen it gives off a mylohyoid branch, which pierces the sphenomandibular ligament and runs downwards and forwards between the ramus and the medial pterygoid to provide the motor nerve supply to the mylohyoid muscle and the anterior belly of the digastric muscle. The mylohyoid nerve provides a cutaneous branch which gives sensory innervation to a small region of skin overlying the point of the chin. In 10 per cent of cadavers examined by Sicher, a twig from the sensory branch enters the mandible in the mental region and may participate in the innervation of the mandibular incisor teeth. The inferior dental nerve then passes along the mandibular canal to provide at least most of the nerve supply to all the teeth on that side of the lower jaw. At the mental foramen, which is usually situated below the apex of the lower second premolar or less commonly below and between the apices of the lower first and second premolars, the nerve divides, one branch continuing in the canal as the *incisive nerve* to supply the first premolar, canine and incisor teeth. It is normal for some cross-innervation to take place between the right and left incisive nerves in this region, this usually extending only to the central incisor on the opposite side, but occasionally to the lateral also. The other branch, the *mental nerve,* emerges from the mental foramen to supply the mucous membrane and skin of the lower lip and chin and the buccal and labial gingivae associated with the mandibular first premolar, canine and incisor teeth.

The mandibular plexus

Carter and Keen (1971) reported that there may be a nerve plexus in the cancellous bone of the mandible lateral to the molar roots and inferior dental canal. It is possible that the lower teeth may be innervated from this mandibular plexus via twigs supplied by the long buccal, lingual and inferior dental nerves. Rood (1976, 1977) has made further comments on this nerve plexus, particularly in relation to innervation of the incisor teeth.

The auriculotemporal nerve

This nerve is of dental significance because it innervates the largest of the salivary glands. It arises by two roots which embrace the middle meningeal artery and then unite, being situated medial to and then behind the condyle of the mandible to supply the temporomandibular joint and the parotid gland. From there it passes upwards in the substance of the gland to the upper border where it divides to supply the skin of the upper half of the pinna and the anterior half of the external auditory meatus via its auricular branch, and part of the skin of the scalp by its cutaneous branch. The parasympathetic fibres, which form the secretomotor supply for the parotid gland, are picked up from the otic ganglion.

REFERENCES AND FURTHER READING

Adatia A. K. and Gehring E. N. (1971) Proprioceptive innervation of the tongue. *J. Anat.* **110,** 215.

Barker B. C. W. (1971) Dissection of regions of interest to the dentist from a medial approach. *Aust. Dent. J.* **16,** 163.

Barker B. C. W. and Davies P. L. (1972) The applied anatomy of the pterygomandibular space. *J. Oral Surg.* **10,** 43.

Barker B. C. W. and Lockett B. C. (1972) Multiple canals in the rami of the mandible. *Oral Surg.* **34,** 384.

Bowsher D. (1980) Central mechanisms of orofacial pain. *Br. J. Oral Surg.* **17,** 185.

Carter R. B. and Keen E. N. (1971) The intramandibular course of the inferior alveolar nerve. *J. Anat.* **108,** 433.

Jeffries C. N. (1944) The inferior alveolar injection for fillings. *Br. Dent. J.* **77,** 152.

Kay L. W. (1974) Some anthropologic investigations of interest to oral surgeons. *Int. J. Oral Surg.* **3,** 363.

Roberts G. D. D. and Harris M. (1973) Neurapraxia of the mylohyoid nerve and submental analgesia. *Br. J. Oral Surg.* **11,** 110.

Rood J. P. (1976) The analgesia and innervation of mandibular teeth. *Br. Dent. J.* **140,** 237.

Rood J. P. (1977) The nerve supply of the mandibular incisor region. *Br. Dent. J.* **143,** 227.

Sicher H. and DuBrul E. L. (1975) *Oral Anatomy,* 6th ed. St Louis, Mosby.

Stewart D. and Wilson S. L. (1928) Regional anaesthesia and innervation of the teeth. *Lancet* **215,** 809.

Chapter 10

INFILTRATION ANALGESIA

The principle of infiltration analgesia is the injection of an analgesic solution very near the actual area to be treated and relying upon the solution diffusing or infiltrating to the sensory nerves so that the conduction of pain impulses is prevented. In the case of a tooth, analgesia is achieved by the solution spreading from the adjacent soft tissues into the bone to reach the nerve fibres leaving the apex.

The main types of infiltration injections are:

1. Submucous and supra- or paraperiosteal.
2. Subperiosteal.
3. Intraligamentary or intraligamental.
4. Intraosseous, including intraseptal.
5. Papillary.

However, when speaking of an infiltration injection one usually refers to the supra-periosteal type and, as this is by far the most frequently used form of local analgesia, the technique is described in some detail.

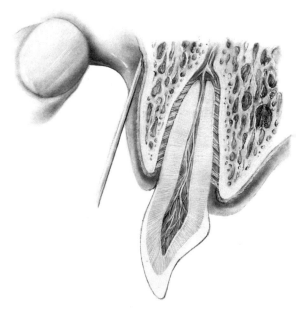

Fig. 10.1. Needle in position for supraperiosteal injection.

SUBMUCOUS AND SUPRAPERIOSTEAL INFILTRATION ANALGESIA

These two types of infiltration injection are very similar. A submucous injection, as its name implies, is the deposition of the analgesic into the submucous tissues just below the surface of the oral epithelium, and a supraperiosteal injection is the deposition of the solution in close approximation to the external surface of the periosteum. It is, of course, desirable in all supraperiosteal injections, where one wishes to achieve analgesia of a tooth, to deposit the solution as near to the apex as possible (*Fig.* 10.1). Thus these two techniques are, in practice, the same when their purpose is to produce analgesia of a tooth. However, this is not so

when infiltrating, for example, beneath the buccal mucosa of the cheek to achieve analgesia of the long buccal nerve. In this situation the injection is given submucosally and it would be inaccurate to term it a supraperiosteal injection.

The efficiency of an infiltration depends on the permeability of the tissues, in particular the bone, through which the analgesic solution has to pass (*Fig.* 10.2). Therefore in the whole of the maxilla, where the bone is relatively permeable and the outer cortical plate thin, an infiltration injection is nearly always effective. The only two situations where difficulty may sometimes be experienced are in the maxillary canine region where the long root passes into fairly dense and thick bone, and in the upper first molar region, where the bone over the apices of

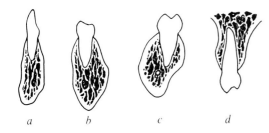

Fig. 10.2. Cross-section of the jaws to show the thickness of bone overlying the apices. *a,* Lower incisor region. *b,* Lower premolar region. *c,* Lower third molar region. *d,* Upper premolar region.

the buccal roots, particularly the mesial, is thickened by the base of the zygomatic process.

In the mandible the story is entirely different because the outer cortical plate of bone is much denser and thicker than that of the maxilla, particularly on the buccal aspects of the teeth from the canine back, thus making infiltration analgesia for the permanent lower molars and premolars unlikely to succeed. The bone of the floor of the incisive fossae, which are situated on the outer aspect of the mandible below the lateral incisors and canines, is relatively permeable, many foramina being present. These allow the solution deposited in these areas to diffuse through the outer cortical plate and into the cancellous bone where it spreads rapidly to the apices of the incisors and more slowly to the canines.

Technique of supraperiosteal infiltration
The whole of the injection technique must be directed towards administering the analgesic painlessly and efficiently and at the same time taking every precaution to avoid unnecessary complications.

Position the patient correctly in the chair
Always have the chair leaning backwards when an injection is to be administered, so as to keep the patient's head as low as possible, an angle of 30° to the vertical being about the minimum which is acceptable. This is to reduce the likelihood of syncope because the lower the patient's head then the less chance there is of a faint occurring. Indeed, if the patient is in the horizontal position it is almost impossible for him to

faint. It is interesting to note that in the days when amputations had to be carried out without general anaesthesia, patients, who were always operated on in the prone position, practically never lost consciousness.

Loading of the syringe
First, prepare the syringe to receive the cartridge as described for the various different types in Chapter 5, but leave the needle cover in place. Never use a cartridge if part of the contents have already been used on a previous patient, because it could be contaminated.

For most infiltrations a needle of gauge 30 and 1 in (25 mm) long is satisfactory. Next, warm the solution in the cartridge to body temperature. This is important because the plunger of the syringe will operate more smoothly on a cartridge which has been warmed. This simplifies the injection technique because it avoids the need for excessive pressure which may result in the sudden injection of the analgesic, again causing pain. Another possible advantage may be the avoidance of discomfort to the patient if a very cold solution is injected, although Rood (1977) reported that patients were unaware of temperature sensation if injected solutions were between 20 and 30 °C, results confirming the earlier work of Oikarinen et al. (1975).

The diaphragm of the cartridge, which will be penetrated by the needle, is now disinfected by one of the methods discussed in Chapter 6 and then the cartridge is inserted into the syringe. This should always be loaded and kept out of sight of the patient. Seeing the syringe would make many apprehensive and some will actually faint before the injection is given. By having the nurse pass the syringe to you from behind the patient at the appropriate moment, and reassuring him when necessary throughout the injection, psychological trauma will be reduced to a minimum and the chance of fainting greatly decreased. Should one have to reload the syringe then the patient's attention can be distracted by asking him to rinse out.

The adoption of this technique is particularly important with the nervous patient or child, especially when it is the first injection he has ever received, as his whole attitude to dentistry in the ensuing years may well depend upon it.

Method of injection

1. Before proceeding with the actual injection it is important to make certain that a pair of Spencer-Wells artery forceps (*Fig.* 10.3) or a similar instrument is close at hand in case of needle breakage. When a needle breaks, the broken end projecting from the tissues will rapidly disappear from sight, so there is only a very short time available in which to attempt its retrieval.

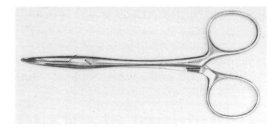

Fig. 10.3. Spencer-Wells artery forceps.

2. Estimate the position of the apex of the tooth because it is desirable to deposit the solution as close to this as possible (*Fig.* 10.4*a*) in order to minimize the distance that the solution has to diffuse. (Reference to the patient's radiographs can be of assistance in this context.)

3. Examine the proposed injection site to check that the tissue is healthy, dry it and then clean it with a non-irritant antiseptic such as a weak iodine solution or chlorhexidine gluconate (Hibitane). The use of an antiseptic on the oral mucosa does not sterilize it but greatly reduces the number of superficial contaminant organisms. After this, apply a surface analgesic and allow 1–2 minutes for this to take effect.

4. Remove the needle guard and test the syringe by ejecting a little fluid to see that the needle is not blocked. Also check that the needle point appears to be sharp and has not been damaged.

5. Pull the surface mucosa taut like a drumskin so that the needle will penetrate the tissues easily (*Fig.* 10.4*b*). Even a very sharp needle will not pass readily into lax tissues and the excess pressure required will cause pain.

If the injection site is one where the insertion of the needle or the initial deposition of the solution is likely to cause pain, then warn the patient of this immediately before inserting the needle. This allows the patient to be prepared

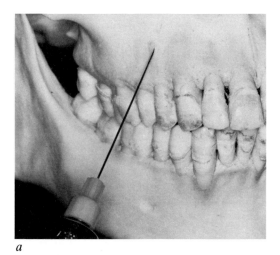

a

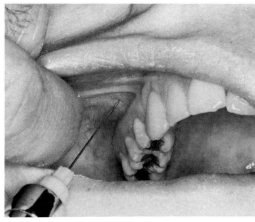

b

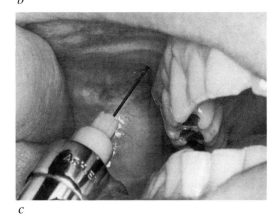

c

Fig. 10.4. Supraperiosteal infiltration. *a,* The needle is positioned so that its point is as nearly opposite the apex of the tooth as possible. *b,* The mucosa is pulled taut prior to inserting the needle. *c,* When the needle point has reached its final position the tissues are relaxed to allow the analgesic to diffuse readily.

for the discomfort and thus reduces the chance of his suddenly moving.

6. As soon as the needle has passed below the surface of the mucosa inject a small amount of solution and wait a few seconds for this to take effect. This will achieve analgesia of the deeper tissues through which the needle has to pass. Care must be taken not to inject while the needle is in the surface epithelium as pain will result because of the forcible separation of the layers of epithelial cells with their relatively abundant innervation. If one injects here it is immediately obvious because a small bleb or weal will be raised on the surface.

7. The needle can now be inserted until its point is as nearly opposite the apex of the tooth as possible. The tissues are relaxed to allow the analgesic to diffuse readily (*Fig.* 10.4*c*) and it is slowly injected after having aspirated to confirm that the needle point is not situated within a blood vessel. The speed of the injection should be at a maximum rate of 2 ml per minute. If injected too rapidly, the tissues are traumatized and this will result in 'after-pain'.

The quantity of analgesic required usually varies between 0·5 and 2 ml per tooth, depending on such factors as the bone structure of the patient, his susceptibility to local analgesics, the operative procedure to be carried out, and the tooth involved. Thus 2 ml will be required for the extirpation of the pulp of an upper molar, whereas 0·8 ml will prove adequate for cutting a simple cavity on an upper premolar, and only 0·2 ml will be needed to achieve local analgesia of the soft tissues.

One must avoid injecting subperiosteally as this will strip the periosteum from the bone and cause prolonged postoperative discomfort (*Fig.* 10.5). Therefore, if the needle strikes the bone it should always be withdrawn a millimetre before injecting.

If, during an injection, the patient starts to feel pain then one should pause until the analgesic already in the tissues has had time to take effect before proceeding. Depending upon the analgesic used, an infiltration injection will usually be effective within 2 minutes. To be on the safe side, approximately 3½–4 minutes should be allowed, and if analgesia has failed to take effect within 6–8 minutes then the injection must be deemed a failure and the cause for this ascertained before a further one is given.

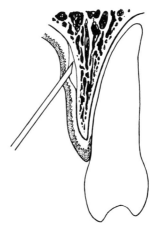

Fig. 10.5. A subperiosteal injection causing elevation of the mucoperiosteum.

When a buccal or labial infiltration is used on any maxillary tooth or on the mandibular incisors (*Fig.* 10.6) it will normally produce complete pulpal analgesia, thus permitting any

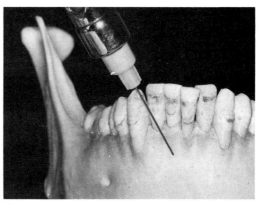

a

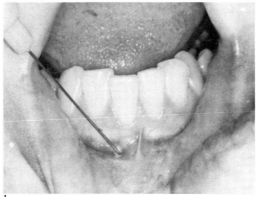

b

Fig. 10.6. Infiltration analgesia for the mandibular incisors.

conservative procedure, including pulpal extirpation. It will also provide soft-tissue analgesia on the outer aspects of the teeth. Where maxillary teeth are to be extracted or surgery of the palatal soft tissues performed, then a palatal injection will also be required. For extraction of mandibular incisors a further infiltration injection is needed on the lingual aspect. If analgesia of the mandibular premolars or molars proves necessary then a nerve block injection should be used. For extraction of these teeth analgesia of the surrounding soft tissues must be obtained by blocking of the long buccal nerve, the lingual nerve usually being blocked at the same time as the inferior dental.

Variation of technique with site

In certain sites particular care is required to avoid unnecessary pain during injections. Examples of these are:

1. The labial aspect of the upper incisors where the base of the nose limits the available tissue into which the fluid can diffuse.

2. The buccal aspect of the upper first molar, due to the malar buttress which is formed by the base of the zygomatic process of the maxilla. This extends particularly over the mesiobuccal root of the molar and leaves very little soft tissue to hold the solution. To overcome this the analgesic can be deposited on either side of the buttress, that is just behind the second premolar and over the distobuccal root of the first molar.

3. The palate, particularly in the anterior region. This is discussed more fully in Chapter 11.

4. The labial aspect of the lower incisors, because of the attachment of the mentalis and the depressor labii inferioris muscles to the underlying mandible.

Thus the use of surface analgesics in these sites is more important and the speed of injection must be far slower. Indeed, whilst in the upper second molar region it may not be necessary to pause during the administration of the analgesic, if one requires to achieve analgesia of several upper anterior teeth painlessly it is often best to infiltrate a few drops of solution and wait 1–2 minutes for soft-tissue analgesia before proceeding with the main injections.

SUBPERIOSTEAL INFILTRATION ANALGESIA

Some authorities advocate the use of subperiosteal injections as opposed to the supraperiosteal technique for the prevention of pain during routine dental treatment as this deposits the solution closer to the apex of the tooth. However, there would seem to be little justification for this for the following reasons:

1. The powerful local analgesics now available will readily pass through the periosteum and it is quite rare for a supraperiosteal infiltration to fail.

2. The injection of a solution subperiosteally must elevate the periosteum from the underlying bone to which it is quite firmly bound. This invariably causes pain at the time of injection and also almost always results in postoperative discomfort, as anyone who has experienced this injection will verify.

One of the few situations in which it is sometimes impossible to avoid injecting subperiosteally is in the anterior part of the palate.

INTRALIGAMENTARY ANALGESIA

This is achieved by injecting an analgesic solution directly into the periodontal membrane of the tooth.

Uses

Originally this technique was introduced specifically for the extraction of teeth in haemophiliacs and patients suffering from similar disorders. Here it is essential to avoid regional analgesia because of the risk of haemorrhage into the deeper tissues. In the case of the inferior dental nerve block, dangerous bleeding into the pterygomandibular region is liable to occur and this might track down into the tissue spaces of the neck to cause fatal respiratory obstruction. Similarly, it is highly desirable to avoid a supraperiosteal injection because of the very extensive haematoma which is likely to arise. By using an intraperiodontal injection, one is merely traumatizing the periodontal membrane which is going to be damaged and partially removed in any case.

More recently much finer needles of gauge 30 have become available and the clinical impression is that if these needles are inserted in the periodontal membrane to a depth of only about 2 mm then no permanent damage is done to that structure. Hence intraligamentary analgesia may be used when conservative treatment is planned for a tooth. The technique is also useful when there is difficulty in obtaining analgesia, as frequently intraligamental injections are successful when other methods have failed. This type of injection has the advantage of minimizing the amount of soft-tissue anaesthesia which occurs when compared with other types of injections. It has largely eliminated the need for the specialized intraosseous injection which did have special indications.

The reduction in the amount of soft-tissue analgesia obtained with the intraligamentary injection applies to both the limited area obtained with an infiltration injection and to more extensive analgesia, such as involves the tongue when an inferior dental nerve block is administered. Patients, particularly children, find the loss of soft-tissue sensation one of the more unpleasant aspects of dentistry and are often, initially at least, scared by this. There is also the risk that they may bite or burn their lip or cheek because they cannot feel it.

Another indication for the intraligamentary injection is to provide analgesia for the extraction of teeth prior to the fitting of an immediate replacement denture. Here the complete lack of distension of soft tissue by the analgesic solution such as occurs with an infiltration injection is of great value. Little difficulty should be experienced in fitting the denture as any alteration in the tissue morphology will be minimal.

Technique

A special intraligamental syringe is used with a gauge 30 short needle. Prior to injecting it is necessary to check that the gingival margin of the tooth is healthy and clean, using a rubber cup to remove debris from the gingival crevice and dental floss soaked in an antiseptic such as 0·1 per cent hexetidine (Oraldene, Warner) to clean interdentally.

The needle is inserted parallel with the long axis of the root of the tooth to a depth of about 2 mm until it contacts the alveolar bone. Then

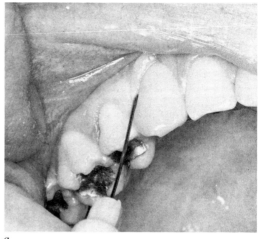

a

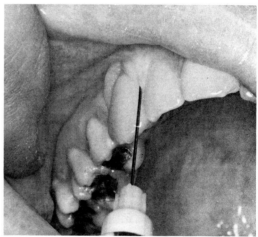

b

Fig. 10.7. Intraligamentary injections for the maxillary canine.

0·2 ml of solution is injected over a period of 30 seconds. This volume is necessary for each root of the tooth, maxillary molars requiring three injections and mandibular molars two. If complete analgesia is not obtained then the injections may be repeated (*Fig.* 10.7). Usually the injections are made on the buccal or labial aspect of the tooth as access is easier, but if the injections are to be repeated then they may be given on the lingual or palatal aspect. The palatal roots of maxillary molars do require palatal injections. Not more than 0·4 ml of solution should be injected for each root, and ideally less as the increased volume of solution injected into the confined space of the periodontal membrane is likely to traumatize the tissues. This is not so important if the tooth is to be extracted but may be critical when the tooth is being conserved. The period of analgesia usually lasts 30–45 minutes, and the onset of analgesia is generally very rapid.

Disadvantages

The technique should not be used when infection is present at the injection site. Occasionally discomfort may occur after the analgesia produced by the injection wears off, but this is usually due to the operator injecting too rapidly or using too great a volume of solution.

INTRAOSSEOUS INJECTIONS

The intraosseous technique is the injection of an analgesic solution into the inner or cancellous portion of the bone, through which it readily diffuses to the apices of the teeth (*Fig.* 10.8). A path for the needle is usually made by drilling through the cortical bone.

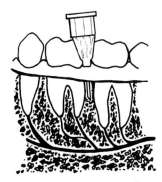

Fig. 10.8. An intraosseous injection in which the solution passes directly into the cancellous bone. The hub should be pressed against the mucosa to prevent back-flow of the anaesthetic.

Uses

The indications for the use of intraosseous injections are now of secondary importance, as the intraligamentary technique usually achieves the same aims and is preferable because it is simpler and does not involve any drilling of the cortical bone prior to injection.

Injection technique

Before administering an intraosseous injection the patient should be warned that it will momentarily increase his heart rate. This is because the vasoconstrictor passes rapidly from the cancellous bone into the bloodstream.

The site at which the drill will enter the tissues is cleaned and a surface antiseptic applied. Analgesia of the tissues through which the drill will pass is then achieved by infiltration of a small amount of solution. The safest method is the *intraseptal approach,* where the injection is made interdentally about 4 mm from the tip of the papilla. An alternative method is to drill through the bone near the apices of the teeth, but this has the grave disadvantage of risking damage to the roots of the teeth and structures such as the inferior dental nerve.

Penetration of the outer cortical plate of bone

This may be achieved by several methods:

1. A round bur, slightly larger than the needle, can be used, but this will not always result in a straight hole through the bone, as the bur may wander.

2. Alternatives are the Beutelrock and the spiral-twist drills which are used in a contra-angle handpiece when employed in the posterior region (*Fig.* 10.9). The only disadvantage of this technique is that the drills are relatively long and flexible, and hence liable to fracture. If this occurs then some difficulty may be experienced in removing the broken portion without risking damage to the adjacent teeth.

3. A third method is to use the special drill designed by E. J. van den Berg. It will be seen that this consists of a twist drill, approximately 5 mm long, incorporating a metal stop which prevents the penetration of the drill into the tissues beyond this depth. An advantage of this method is that special needles are manufactured which correspond in size with the twist drill (*Fig.* 10.10), thus reducing the likelihood of backflow of the analgesic through the opening of the bone at the time of injection. The only disadvantage is that occasionally the outer cortical plate of bone may be thicker than the maximum depth of 5 mm to which the drill is able to penetrate.

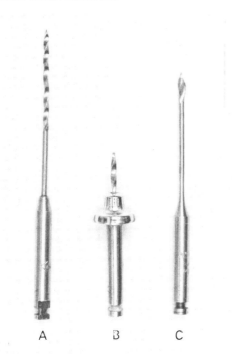

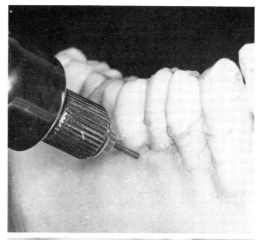

a

Fig. 10.9. Various drills used for penetrating the cortical plate of the bone. *a,* Spiral-twist drill. *b,* van den Berg drill. *c,* Beutelrock drill.

Having chosen the drill, which must have been carefully sterilized, it is passed through the outer cortical plate interdentally at an angle of approximately 45° to the long axis of the tooth and then withdrawn (*Figs.* 10.11*b,* 10.12*b*).

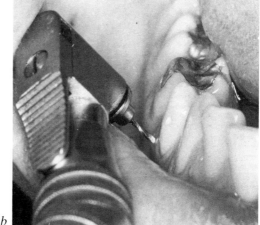

b

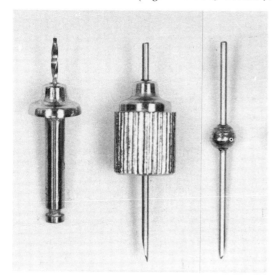

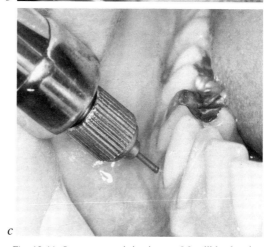

c

Fig. 10.11. Intraosseous injection. *a,* Mandible showing site of injection. *b,* van den Berg drill in a contra-angle handpiece penetrating the cortical plate. *c,* Matching needle being inserted into the bone. When fully seated the hub will press firmly against the soft tissues to ensure a seal.

Fig. 10.10. Matching van den Berg drill and needles.

Immediately after this, and without disturbing the mucoperiosteum in any way by movement of the fingers and thus 'losing' the hole in the bone, the needle is inserted (*Figs*. 10.11*a*, *c*, 10.12*a*, *c*) and pressed firmly into place.

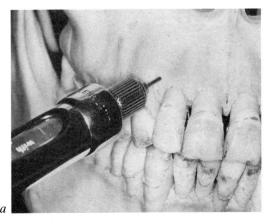

a

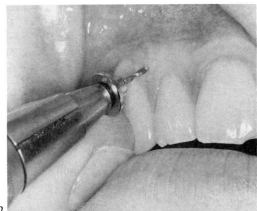

b

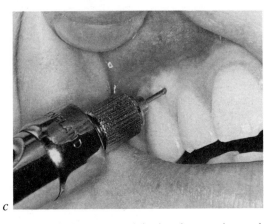

c

Fig. 10.12. Intraosseous injection for anterior teeth where the van den Berg drill is used in a straight handpiece.

When the van den Berg drill is used the matched needles should be employed. These have an advantage over ordinary needles in that their tips are blunt and rounded, thus allowing them to pass easily through the hole. An ordinary sharp needle point tends to 'snag' on the sides of the channel drilled through the cortical plate. When an ordinary needle is employed, then it should be a short one with a wide bore used in a long hub to prevent undue penetration of the needle into the cancellous bone. Because the needle does not fit the hole accurately, a rubber seal (*Fig.* 10.13) should be placed on it to prevent the back-flow of the analgesic solution at the time of injection. Only 0·5 ml of analgesic is normally required. No pressure is needed to deposit the solution as it passes easily into the cancellous bone, analgesia being almost instantaneous.

When used with children under the age of 10–11 for treatment of the lower first permanent molar, it is not generally necessary to drill through the bone; firm pressure with a short 25-gauge needle in a long hub is adequate to pass through the thin interseptal bone on either side of the tooth.

As the analgesia achieved will often only be of 10 minutes' duration, and frequently less, it is important to start operative procedures as quickly as possible after the injection.

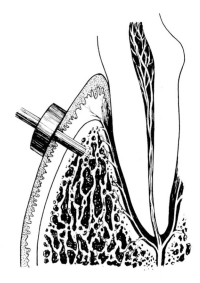

Fig. 10.13. Use of a rubber seal to prevent back-flow of analgesic solution during injection.

Advantages of the technique

1. Rapidity of onset, analgesia being obtained in a matter of seconds.

2. Avoidance of soft-tissue analgesia and swelling.

3. As already mentioned, it may succeed where other techniques fail.

Disadvantages of the technique

1. The technique is rather more complex than a supraperiosteal infiltration, it being desirable to have a special set of standardized drills and needles.

2. The duration of analgesia is usually not longer than 10 minutes and often only 2–3 minutes due to the rapid diffusion of the solution through the highly vascular cancellous bone and into the bloodstream. This may occasionally be advantageous.

3. Due to the rapid absorption into the bloodstream it is apt to affect the patient far more at the time of injection than a supraperiosteal infiltration and thus they should be warned of this. Also as stated on p. 26 when commenting on the work of Cannell et al. (1975), care must be taken not to exceed a safe circulating level of analgesic because of the vascularity of cancellous bone.

4. The intraosseous technique is not easy to apply in the molar region because of difficulty of access, a curved needle being desirable.

5. By injecting into the bone there is a slight risk of causing infection or osteomyelitis, especially if a very careful sterilization technique is not employed.

PAPILLARY INFILTRATION

This method is based upon the injection of the analgesic solution into the soft tissues of the interdental papilla.

Technique

The interdental papilla which is to be the site of the first injection is dried, cleaned with an antiseptic, and a surface analgesic applied.

After this has taken effect, the needle, of 25 gauge and 1 in (25 mm) length, preferably used with a long hub for rigidity, is inserted into the centre of the papilla at a level at which this soft tissue is attached to the underlying periosteum. Where periodontal disease has caused pocketing with detachment of the papillae, then the syringe needle will have to be inserted further from the gingival margin so that it still enters the attached gingiva. A small quantity of analgesic, usually not more than 0·25 ml, is slowly administered, considerable pressure being required. As the solution is injected there is blanching of the surrounding tissues which gradually spreads to involve the adjacent papillae (*Fig.* 10.14). When this occurs, it indicates that the solution has reached these papillae and their analgesia is achieved. There is then no need for further injection at the first site. The needle is now transferred to the adjacent papilla and the

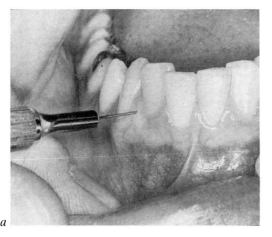
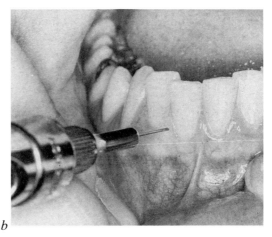

a   *b*

Fig. 10.14. A syringe with a long hub and a short needle being used for serial papillary injections.

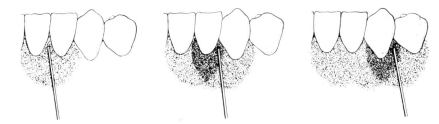

Fig. 10.15. Serial papillary injections in which the shading indicates the spread of analgesia to the adjacent papillae prior to their injection.

process repeated until, by means of several injections, analgesia of the whole area which one requires to operate upon is obtained (*Fig.* 10.15). This technique depends upon the considerable pressure exerted within the soft tissues by the solution in order to achieve the effective spread of analgesia.

Advantages and uses

The technique is of particular use when carrying out a gingivectomy or any other operation of a similar nature because a high degree of haemostasis is achieved, and this makes the performance of the operation and the subsequent placing of a pack far simpler. Only a very small quantity of analgesic is required and the area involved is minimal. Little after-pain occurs due to the analgesic, as most of the tissues into which it was injected will have been removed.

Disadvantages

A relatively large number of injections are required by comparison with any other technique and thus it is time-consuming. It is difficult to perform on the lingual aspect of the mandible and the initial injection tends to be painful because of the pressure involved in injecting into a firm tissue which is tightly bound down to underlying bone by fibrous tissue.

INTRAFOLLICULAR ANAESTHESIA

W. H. Wall (1985) has described an infiltration technique, which he terms 'intrafollicular anaesthesia', for producing analgesia for the removal of impacted mandibular third molars. The needle is inserted into the intraseptal region via the interdental papilla and using a gradually increasing pressure, about 0·5 ml of local anaesthetic solution is injected so that it reaches the underlying bone to enter the follicular space which surrounds the unerupted tooth. A 25-gauge needle is used and this may be inserted to a depth of 1–2 cm to enter the follicular space.

Dr Wall considers the injection is equivalent to an intravenous injection and therefore the concentration of epinephrine (adrenaline) should not exceed 1 : 100 000. The onset of analgesia is very rapid as this injection region is relatively vascular. He reports that this technique works well even with acutely abscessed teeth, but warns against injecting into abscess cavities. Certainly this must not be done because the anaesthetic solution would probably spread any infection present. Apparently with the intrafollicular injections, additional injections are administered in the region innervated by the long buccal nerve, submucosally in the retromolar pad area, and sometimes these are supplemented with an inferior dental nerve block. The more conventional routine for the removal of an impacted lower third molar under local analgesia would require an inferior dental nerve block to anaesthetize the inferior dental and lingual nerves, and a buccal infiltration to anaesthetize the fibres of the long buccal nerve. Possibly the intrafollicular injection is of value when there is difficulty in achieving satisfactory analgesia for the removal of an impacted tooth using the standard injections.

JET INJECTION

An alternative to depositing an analgesic solution hypodermically be means of a needle is the use of a jet injector. With this instrument a jet of local analgesic of far finer diameter than a 30-gauge needle is fired at the soft tissues with sufficient force to penetrate them.

The advantages of this technique are that it is rapid and virtually painless. However, only a relatively limited amount of solution can be fired into the soft tissues without causing undue trauma. Moreover, if the injector is moved during firing or used on mobile unattached tissues then the mucosa will be cut (*Fig.* 14.13). Thus the injection should ideally be made onto attached tissues, but a difficulty which arises here is that these can accept only a limited amount of solution before tissue damage occurs.

The jet injector is of particular use in obtaining analgesia in regions such as the hard palate, where a conventional injection technique tends to be painful. Jet injection is also of value when superficial analgesia is required for tasks such as extracting loose teeth, for localized surgery or prior to taking a deep subgingival impression for crown and bridgework. More recently, Lambrianidis et al. (1980) have reported on the use of jet injection as the sole means of inducing analgesia for extracting firm permanent teeth in adults. Lignocaine of up to 50 per cent strength was used with a high rate of success and it was planned to try even more concentrated analgesic solutions. This experimental work may lead to the successful use of jet injection for inducing pulpal analgesia for all types of routine dentistry.

The area of analgesia achieved depends on the instrument used. In the case of the Panjet, the dosage of 0·04 ml cannot be varied and will achieve a maximum area of analgesia approximately 1 cm in diameter. In the case of the Syrijet the dosage may be varied between 0·01 and 0.2 ml according to need.

As reported on p. 50, the Med-E-Jet, which can inject a single dose of up to 1 ml, has been used successfully to give inferior dental blocks. The administration of these blocks by jet injection was much more comfortable for the patients than for those who were given the normal aspirating hypodermic syringe. However, these jet injection blocks were given during a research project and further studies need to be done before the use of a jet injector can be considered as a routine method for nerve block injections.

CAUSES OF FAILURE OF INFILTRATION ANALGESIA

1. Deposition of analgesic solution in the wrong area during a supraperiosteal injection

It should always be placed supraperiosteally and as nearly over the apex of the tooth as possible. This can be assessed from the position of the crown. A common error is to infiltrate too far away from bone or too deeply into soft tissue, when the solution is liable to pass intramuscularly which, apart from causing failure of analgesia, will also result in after-pain (*Fig.* 10.16).

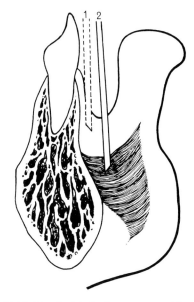

Fig. 10.16. Needle 1 is in the correct position for infiltration in the mandibular incisor region. Needle 2 is too deep and too far away from the surface of the bone, so that it has entered a muscle. The bevel of the needle is also incorrect as the solution will not be directed towards the bone.

2. Wrong assessment of the dosage required

The amount of analgesic solution must be assessed correctly, the dosage required depending on the thickness and density of the bone through which it has to pass. This varies with:

a. The patient. If patients are well-built and have a heavy bone structure then a larger dosage will be required than if they are small and frail. Males tend to need more analgesic than females.

b. The local anatomy. A larger dosage is required, for instance, over a maxillary canine, where the bone is relatively thick and the root lying comparatively deeply, as opposed to an upper second premolar, where the root is more superficial and the overlying bone far thinner.

3. Incorrect choice of analgesic solution

Failure to choose the correct analgesic solutions for the work in hand accounts for many failures. Thus whereas the use of practically any analgesic solution will achieve soft-tissue analgesia, a fairly potent drug is required for cavity preparations, and for pulpal analgesia a still more powerful local analgesic is necessary. Although lignocaine alone will be adequate for soft-tissue analgesia of short duration, failure will frequently occur if it is used prior to cutting dentine. Here a solution such as carbocaine or prilocaine will usually prove adequate and its potency will be increased if a vasoconstrictor is added. At the present time the most profound analgesia is probably produced by a combination of 2 per cent lignocaine with 1 : 80 000 adrenaline. Rood and Sowray have reported on the experimental clinical use of 5 per cent lignocaine with 1 : 80 000 adrenaline and obtained successful analgesia from this solution in many instances when 2 per cent lignocaine with the same vasoconstrictor has been ineffective (Rood and Sowray, 1980). This 5 per cent lignocaine solution for dental use is not yet available commercially.

4. Incorrect choice of technique

Analgesia which may be fully adequate for an extraction may be of insufficient depth for routine conservation, and pulp extirpation demands more profound analgesia than either conservation or extraction. Apicectomy also requires a deep level of analgesia, possibly because of the infection usually present around the apex of the tooth. Where deep prolonged analgesia is required, regional analgesia will often prove more satisfactory than an infiltration technique.

5. Incorrect technique in presence of inflammation or infection

An analgesic is usually ineffective in the presence of inflamed tissue, the reason for this being unknown. It is thought that the altered pH of inflamed tissues may inactivate the solution, but another factor could be the increased irritability of the nerve fibres. Further theories have been discussed in Chapter 7 (*see* p. 68. Where inflammation is present an infiltration injection should be avoided and either a regional nerve block used or a general anaesthetic administered. The latter is usually the method of choice for extractions in these circumstances.

6. Intravascular injection

Although this complication may occur during any infiltration injection, it is particularly likely to happen when injecting in the upper second or third molar regions or when giving an inferior dental block. If this occurs one may see a sudden pallor of the face and often the patient will either feel faint or lose consciousness. Although an aspirating syringe should be used to prevent intravascular injection, if one inserts the needle and injects very slowly then the blood vessels usually contract before the needle reaches them, thus avoiding this complication. As soon as the patient shows any sign that an intravascular injection is being given, the needle should be partially withdrawn to remove it from the lumen of the blood vessel and aspiration repeated before administering any further analgesic solution.

7. Variation in individual tolerance to the analgesic solution

Individuals vary considerably in their degree of resistance to the achievement and duration of local analgesia. Thus one may have a particular patient who never requires more than 0·5 ml for any infiltration injection, whereas another may invariably require at least 2 ml. Similarly, the duration of analgesia may vary between individuals from 20 minutes to 6 hours with the same amount of analgesic. Therefore it is desirable to note on the patient's record card the type, quantity and strength of analgesic used. This is particularly important when the patient varies considerably from the norm.

8. Variation in the pain threshold of individuals and even the same individual on different occasions

The degree of pain tolerance varies very widely with different individuals, and the sensation which one may interpret as pain another would merely consider discomfort. Obviously in the former a far deeper level of analgesia is required. To lower the pain threshold pre-medication is sometimes indicated and this may be administered as described in Chapter 13 on 'Sedation Techniques.' The tolerance of any one individual varies quite considerably from time to time due to such factors as systemic disease, domestic worries, tiredness or hunger.

REFERENCES

Lambrianidis T., Rood J. P. and Sowray J. H. (1980) Dental analgesia by jet injection. *Br. J. Oral Surg.* **17,** 227.

Lilienthal B. (1975) A clinical appraisal of intraosseous dental anaesthesia. *Oral Surg.* **39,** 692.

Oikarinen V. J., Ylipaavalniemi P. and Evers H. (1975) Pain and temperature sensations related to local analgesia. *Int. J. Oral Surg.* **4,** 151.

Rood J. P. (1977) The temperature of local anaesthetic solutions. *J. Dent.* **5,** 213.

Rood J. P. and Sowray J. H. (1980) Clinical experience with 5 per cent lignocaine solution. *J. Dent.* **8,** 128.

Wall W. H. (1985) Intrafollicular anaesthesia for the removal of impacted teeth. In: Derrick D. D. (ed.), *The Dental Annual*. Bristol, Wright, pp. 217–229.

Chapter 11

ANALGESIA OF THE PALATE

LOCAL ANATOMY

The nerve supply of this region is derived from the maxillary division of the trigeminal nerve.

The long sphenopalatine nerve (*Fig.* 11.1) supplies the mucoperiosteum, alveolar process and gingivae of the anterior part of the palate. It gains access to the palate by means of the incisive canal.

The greater palatine nerve (*Fig.* 11.5*a*) reaches the palate by passing through the greater palatine foramen which is situated medially to the second or third molar. It supplies the mucoperiosteum and alveolar process of the whole of the hard palate posterior to the canine, and in the canine region overlaps with the long sphenopalatine nerve.

The lesser palatine nerves (*Fig.* 9.4) emerge from the lesser palatine foramina which usually lie a little behind the posterior palatine foramen. They supply the mucosa of the soft palate and the uvula.

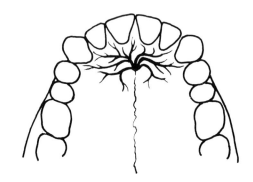

Fig. 11.1. The long sphenopalatine nerve emerging from the incisive foramen.

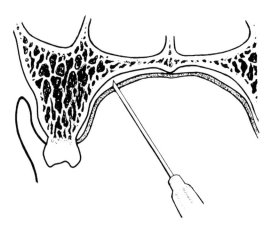

Fig. 11.2. An infiltration injection being given where maximum thickness of soft tissue is available to absorb the analgesic.

TECHNIQUES

Palatal infiltration analgesia

This is the usual method of producing analgesia of the palatal mucosa, particularly in the region of only one or two teeth.

The injection should always be made at the site where the maximum thickness of tissue is available to absorb the analgesic. In the posterior region this is roughly equidistant from the midline and the gingival margins of the teeth, which is at the point of maximum curvature of the palate (*Fig.* 11.2).

The needle, a short one of not less than 27 gauge, is inserted as nearly at right-angles to the

palate as is practicable (*Fig.* 11.3). With care it is possible to avoid injecting subperiosteally by inserting the needle gently until it just touches bone and then withdrawing a little. This prevents the painful elevation of the muco-

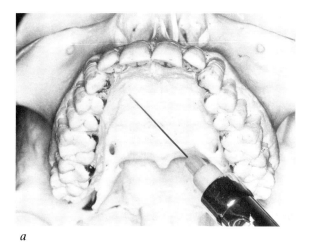
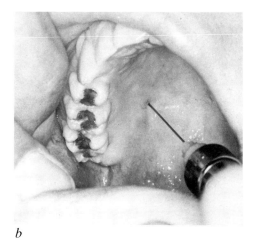

a   *b*

Fig. 11.3. The palatal infiltration injection.

periosteum and also lessens the risk of injecting into the blood vessels which lie close to the bone in this region. A very slow injection is essential, 0·3 ml being administered.

Long sphenopalatine nerve block

Where it is required to achieve analgesia of the palatal mucosa adjacent to the four upper incisors, then it is best to 'block' the long sphenopalatine nerves at, or just before they leave, the incisive fossa. Although this is the main nerve supply to the palatal mucosa behind the six anterior teeth, a 'block' of only this nerve cannot be relied on for the canine region because of overlapping innervation from the greater palatine nerve. The opening of the incisive canal on to the palate is marked by the incisive papilla in the midline and is slightly posterior to the two central incisors. This papilla is extremely sensitive and, unless great care is exercised, a long sphenopalatine nerve block can be very painful. Therefore, a few drops of analgesic solution should be injected initially a little to one side of the papilla (*Fig.* 11.4*a*). After these have taken effect the needle

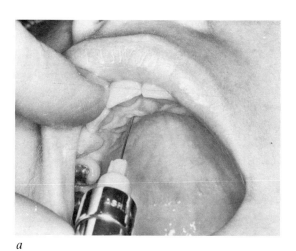
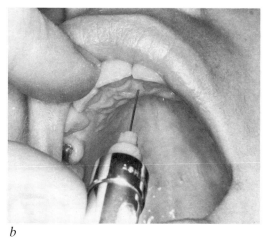

a   *b*

Fig. 11.4. Long sphenopalatine nerve block. *a*, A little solution is infiltrated to one side of the incisive papilla. *b*, The needle is then inserted directly into the papilla.

is inserted just into the incisive papilla at a site exactly on a line midway between the central incisors and parallel to their long axes (*Fig. 11.4b*). A short needle is employed and approximately 0.5 ml of the analgesic solution is injected very slowly.

To obtain analgesia of the palatal mucosa opposite a canine at the same time as the incisor region, an infiltration on the palatal aspect of this tooth will be necessary in addition to the nerve block.

Greater palatine nerve block

The greater palatine foramen through which the nerve passes (*Fig. 11.5a*) is situated medial to the second and third molars, approximately midway between the palatal gingival margins of these teeth and the midline. It opens in an anterior, slightly medial direction. To block the nerve at this point a syringe with a short needle of approximately 27 gauge is used and the foramen approached from the opposite side of the mouth because of the angulation of its opening (*Fig. 11.5b,c*). About 0·25 ml of the analgesic solution should be injected slowly to prevent undue discomfort and avoid lifting the periosteum which invariably causes after-pain. As the fibres of the greater palatine nerve run forwards from the canal, it is best to err a little on the anterior side of the foramen when giving the injection as one will still be certain to obtain the analgesia required and at the same time avoid the unpleasant condition of having analgesia of the soft palate. This is particularly advisable in patients prone to 'retching', which may occur with this injection. Another advantage of not injecting too far posteriorly is that it minimizes the loss of analgesic solution into the lax tissues of the soft palate where it would be ineffective.

It will be realized from the foregoing that analgesia of the whole of the hard palate on one side can be obtained by a combination of long sphenopalatine and greater palatine nerve blocks.

COMPLICATIONS AND CONTRAINDICATIONS

All palatal injections are normally painful, even when care is exercised, because of the firmness

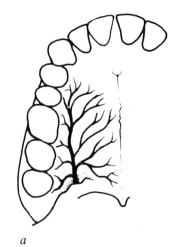

a

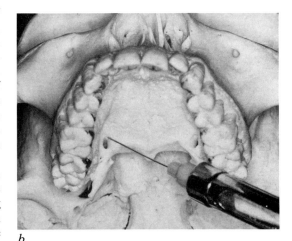

b

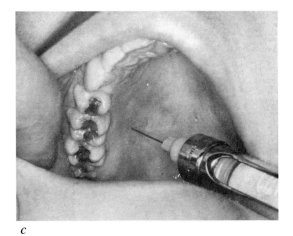

c

Fig. 11.5. *a*, The greater palatine nerve emerging from its foramen. *b*, *c*, The greater palatine nerve block.

of the tissues in this region and their inability to absorb the solution readily. For this reason they should be avoided on young children and nervous patients whenever possible. When they are used in conjunction with a buccal or labial infiltration, it is best to administer this first and then wait for 5 minutes before injecting on the palatal side. In many instances it will be found that the solution has diffused through from the buccal or labial to the palatal aspects and achieved at least some degree of analgesia there, thus rendering the palatal infiltration far less uncomfortable.

A jet injector is simpler, quicker and less painful to use for palatal analgesia than the conventional hypodermic syringe. Care must be taken to keep the injector closely applied to the mucosa and absolutely stationary when firing it in order to minimize the risk of causing unnecessary trauma.

Another technique which may avoid the discomfort of a palatal injection for the extraction of a maxillary deciduous tooth is to give a buccal or labial infiltration and, when this has worked, to administer papillary injections on the same aspect to the two interdental papillae. The solution will diffuse through to the palatal aspect and provide sufficient analgesia without recourse to a palatal injection.

If care is not taken when giving a palatal infiltration, and too much solution is injected rapidly, then detachment of the palatal mucoperiosteum will occur, causing pain and tenderness of the palate which may last for several days.

With palatal block injections it is not advisable to insert the needle beyond the entrance to the foramina. If the needle is passed into the bony canal then there will be the risk of damaging the nerves and vessels which traverse them.

Chapter 12

REGIONAL ANALGESIA

Regional analgesia is the technique used for blocking the passage of pain along the nerve trunk by injecting analgesic solution around it at a site where the nerve is normally unprotected by bone. The blocks used in dental surgery may be considered under those involving:

The maxillary nerve and its branches.
The mandibular nerve and its branches.

THE MAXILLARY NERVE AND ITS BRANCHES

Injections can be used to block the following nerves:

1. The greater and lesser palatine and long sphenopalatine nerves.
2. The posterior superior dental nerve.
3. The middle superior dental nerve.
4. The anterior superior dental nerve, blocked by the infraorbital injection.
5. The maxillary nerve itself.

1. The greater and lesser palatine and long sphenopalatine nerves

The injections for these nerves have already been described in Chapter 11.

2. Posterior superior dental nerve

The posterior superior dental nerve or nerves (*Fig.* 12.1) supply the upper second and third molars, the distobuccal and palatal roots of the first molar, the associated periodontal membranes, the buccal alveolar plate and the neighbouring buccal mucosa. It does not supply the mesiobuccal root of the first molar if the middle

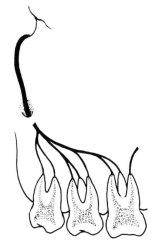

Fig. 12.1. The posterior superior dental nerve. The mesiobuccal root of the first molar is supplied by either the middle or the anterior superior dental nerve.

superior dental nerve is present, or the palatal mucosa. The posterior superior dental nerves pass downwards on the posterior aspect of the maxilla and enter a fine foramen or foramina at the distal aspect of the maxillary tuberosity above and behind the third molar.

Technique
A mirror is used to check that the site is free from infection and then the patient's mouth should be partly closed and relaxed to allow adequate retraction of the cheek. A syringe with a long needle, usually of 27 gauge, should always be used, it being inserted opposite the mesial root of the third molar at the deepest part of the mucogingival fold (*Fig.* 12.2). The needle is now passed inwards, upwards and backwards at an angle of about 45° for approximately

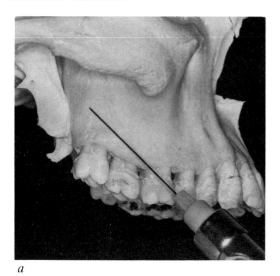

a

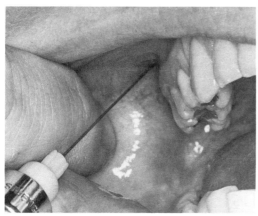

b

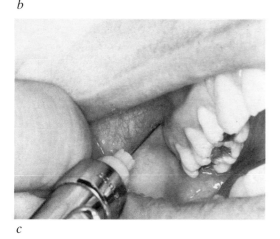

c

Fig. 12.2. Posterior superior dental nerve block showing the needle passing inwards, upwards and backwards at an angle of approximately 45°.

2–2·5 cm, thus passing around the curvature of the posterior aspect of the maxillary tuberosity (*Fig.* 12.2*c*). The needle should on no account be inserted beyond 2·5 cm, as it will then be merely passing away from the nerve and, more important, be liable to enter the pterygoid plexus of veins with resultant haematoma formation. For the same reason the needle should be kept close to the bone throughout its insertion (*Fig.* 12.2*a*), and aspiration should always be performed prior to injecting the solution.

Complications and contraindications

This region is the commonest in which haematoma formation may complicate an injection, the swelling occurring very rapidly and taking several days to disperse with considerable external discoloration of the skin. If one has any doubts as to whether a haematoma is forming, then firm pressure should immediately be applied to the area and maintained for 5 minutes. Some authorities recommend the prescribing of an antibiotic to lessen the risk of the haematoma becoming infected but this is not usually necessary. To reduce the likelihood of haematoma formation the needle should be inserted slowly, pausing from time to time to allow the vasoconstrictor to take effect so that the blood vessels are contracted before the needle reaches them, and injecting continuously as the needle is advanced.

Many consider that the use of the posterior superior dental nerve block is not justified in view of the risks involved, especially when considering the extremely reliable results which can be achieved by the more comfortable and safer infiltration technique.

Maxillary molar block

Adatia (1968) described a technique for the posterior superior dental nerve block which reduced the risk of haematoma formation. The injection numbs all the maxillary molars in that quadrant including the mesiobuccal root of the first molar. He used a 26-gauge needle, 30–42 mm long. Quoting from his description: 'With the patient's mouth half-closed, the cheek is retracted as far as possible. The zygomatic process of the maxilla is palpated and the mucosa in this area is prepared for injection.

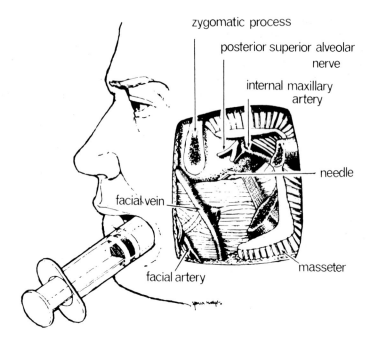

zygomatic process

posterior superior alveolar nerve

internal maxillary artery

needle

facial vein

masseter

facial artery

Fig. 12.3. Diagram to illustrate the posterior superior alveolar nerve and the neighbouring structures in relation to the site of deposition of the local analgesic solution in order to avoid vascular injury. (After Adatia A. K. (1976) *Br. Dent. J.* **140**, 88, by kind permission of the Editor.)

With the cheek still retracted, the bevel of the needle is placed towards the alveolar plate high in the mucobuccal fold just posterior to the zygomatic process of the maxilla. After puncturing the buccal mucosa the needle is advanced upwards, backwards, and inwards for only about 1 cm (*Fig.* 12.3), and the anaesthetic solution is injected. As the solution accumulates just above the buccinator muscle, the attachment of the muscle to the maxilla becomes sharply demarcated by a bulge. After withdrawing the needle a finger is placed over the bulge, which is pushed upwards, backwards, and inwards. At this stage it is convenient to ask the patient to close the mouth, as this allows more room for the finger in the oral vestibule.'

3. Middle superior dental nerve

This nerve is absent in approximately 50 per cent of patients. However, when present it supplies the mesiobuccal root of the upper first molar and both upper premolars. It leaves the infraorbital canal and passes downwards in the anterolateral wall of the antrum to reach the apices of the premolars and the mesiobuccal root of the first molar. Together with the anterior and posterior superior dental nerves it forms what is known as the superior dental plexus or outer nerve loop.

The nerve (*Fig.* 12.4) is blocked at the same time as the anterior superior dental when an infraorbital injection is given, the analgesic

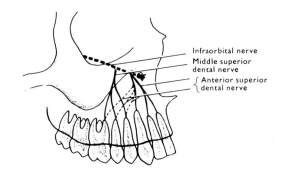

Infraorbital nerve
Middle superior dental nerve
{ Anterior superior
{ dental nerve

Fig. 12.4. The infraorbital nerve showing the anterior and middle superior dental branches. When the middle superior dental nerve is absent the premolars are innervated by fibres from the anterior superior dental nerve, shown in lightly dotted outline.

solution diffusing back along the infraorbital canal to the point where the middle superior dental nerve usually originates. However, if it arises in the posterior part of the canal then it may not be accessible to the analgesic solution, but whatever its anatomical path, its branches are readily reached by an infiltration injection over the teeth they supply and this is usually the method of choice.

4. The infraorbital injection

This injection technique achieves analgesia of the anterior superior dental nerve, which supplies the maxillary incisors and canine, and usually also the middle superior dental nerve which innervates the maxillary premolars and the mesiobuccal root of the first molar. The lateral nasal and superior labial nerves are also affected.

The principle of this injection is the deposition of analgesic solution just inside the infraorbital foramen so that it will diffuse back through the canal to reach the anterior and middle superior dental nerves, the former being given off about 0·5 cm before the outer end of the canal and the latter a variable distance farther back.

Uses

This nerve block is of particular use when carrying out surgery such as gaining access to the maxillary sinus, the removal of a buried upper canine or an apicectomy in the upper anterior region. It is not normally used for routine procedures, but is of value when an infiltration injection has proved ineffective or is contraindicated.

This nerve may be blocked by either an intraoral or an extraoral approach, the latter only being used on rare occasions when access is difficult.

Technique

1. INTRAORAL APPROACH First, the infraorbital foramen is identified. This lies immediately below the pupil of the eye, when the patient is looking straight ahead, and on a line between the pupil and the upper second premolar (*Figs.* 12.5, 12.6*a*). It can be found by palpating the

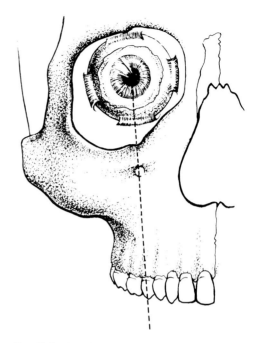

Fig. 12.5. The infraorbital foramen lies on a line joining the upper second premolar and the pupil of the eye when the patient is looking straight ahead.

infraorbital ridge until the infraorbital notch is located, the infraorbital foramen being felt as a shallow depression about 0·5 cm below the notch. The index finger should be kept firmly on this spot, so that it will protect the eye by preventing the needle point from travelling above the foramen. The lip is now retracted by the thumb and the mucosa in the second premolar area is cleaned. A 27-gauge, 1⅝-in (42-mm) needle is passed into the mucobuccal fold adjacent to the second premolar and a little way out from this (*Fig.* 12.6*b*). The needle is then slowly inserted injecting a small amount of solution as it is advanced in a line parallel with the pupil of the eye, the infraorbital notch, and the second premolar, this line usually corresponding with the long axis of the second premolar. When the tip of the needle reaches the infraorbital foramen, the analgesic solution being deposited will be felt by the finger. The needle is then advanced into the foramen for a short distance, aspiration is carried out and the bulk of the solution, about 1·0 ml, is slowly injected, the finger being kept over the foramen to seal it. If the needle is passed a little beyond

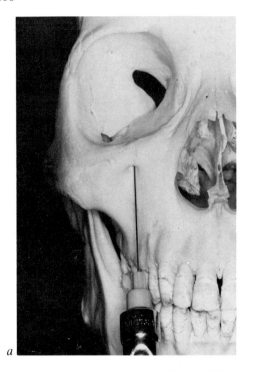

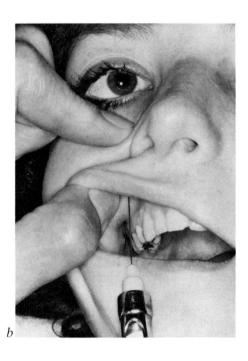

Fig. 12.6. The intraoral infraorbital injection.

this it will strike the upper aspect of the infra-orbital ridge. If the needle has been kept too near the bone it will strike the floor of the canine fossa before travelling far enough and then it must be withdrawn and reinserted farther away from the bone. The maximum depth of insertion of the needle is usually 2 cm. After injection, the solution is gently massaged into the infraorbital foramen.

2. EXTRAORAL APPROACH Where the intraoral technique is contraindicated for any reason, such as infection at the site of insertion of the needle, then an extraoral approach may be made. This is basically similar to the intraoral technique but the distance to be travelled by the needle is considerably less.

First, the skin overlying the injection site is very carefully cleaned. The infraorbital notch is located by palpation and the finger retained there. An imaginary line is drawn down from this to the long axis of the second premolar, as the infraorbital foramen normally lies on this line about 5 mm below the infraorbital ridge. The patient is now told to close the eyes and keep quite still as any sudden movement during

the insertion of the needle might result in damage to the eye. The finger is kept over the infraorbital margin to act as a guard.

The needle is inserted approximately 1 cm below the ridge and passed upwards and inwards at an angle of 45°, keeping the syringe in the same long axis as the line connecting the pupil, infraorbital notch and upper second premolar. The needle is slowly passed into the tissues to a depth of about 1 cm, injecting as it proceeds until the analgesic solution can be felt by the finger being deposited at the foramen (*Fig.* 12.7). After a delay of about 15–20 seconds to obtain local analgesia, the foramen is gently felt for with the needle which is then passed into it for a few millimetres. The finger is pressed firmly over the foramen to seal it and prevent the back-flow of analgesic solution and 1 ml is very slowly deposited, giving ample time for it to diffuse back through the infraorbital canal.

Complications and contraindications

Complications with this injection are rare; however, great care must be taken with steriliz-

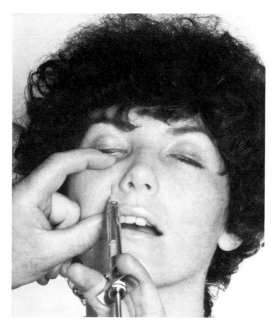

Fig. 12.7. The extraoral infraorbital injection showing the index finger placed above the foramen.

analgesia may not be achieved, hence the need for careful aspiration. Trauma to these vessels can also cause unsightly bruising of the skin which may take as long as 10–14 days to resolve. On rare occasions diplopia may occur due to analgesic entering the orbit as described on p. 152.

5. The maxillary nerve block

The maxillary nerve (*Fig.* 12.8) may be blocked by three different techniques:

1. By the posterior infraorbital injection, the nerve being blocked before it enters the infra-orbital canal by passing a needle up behind the zygomatic surface of the maxilla until it has reached the inferior orbital fissure.

2. By passing a needle up the greater palatine canal to allow the analgesic solution to reach the infraorbital groove.

3. By an external approach.

ation in this region and the technique should never be used if any infection is present; this is because the venous drainage travels back to the cavernous sinus and thus cavernous sinus thrombosis could result. This complication is discussed in Chapter 14.

There is a small risk of entering the anterior facial or infraorbital veins and thus injecting intravenously, with the result that adequate

Indications

This nerve block is a deep one which is difficult to perform and should not be used unless there is a very strong indication for it. The times when this nerve block can be of help are:

a. When analgesia of the entire distribution of the maxillary nerve is required for surgery, such as that involving the antrum or for the removal of a deeply buried upper third molar.

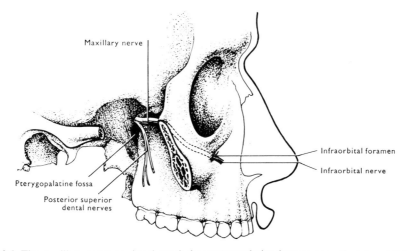

Maxillary nerve

Pterygopalatine fossa

Posterior superior dental nerves

Infraorbital foramen

Infraorbital nerve

Fig. 12.8. The maxillary nerve passing through the pterygopalatine fossa to enter the infraorbital canal.

The bilateral use of this technique will achieve complete analgesia of the maxilla for the extensive surgery required when dealing with lesions such as malignant tumours.

b. Where local nerve blocks, such as the infraorbital or infiltration techniques, are contraindicated because of infection.

c. For diagnostic purposes, particularly when dealing with conditions such as neuralgias, causalgias and tics.

Technique

1. POSTERIOR INFRAORBITAL APPROACH (*Fig.* 12.9) Because of the angulation and depth of insertion necessary, a $1\frac{5}{8}$-in (42-mm) (or longer) needle on a curved or contra-angled hub attachment is used. A piece of sterile rubber dam is placed as a marker on the shaft of the needle 3 cm from the tip.

The mucosa is cleaned thoroughly and the needle inserted over the apices of the second molar and a little distance away from bone in order to clear the zygomatic process. The needle is slowly passed upwards and inwards, the angulation being approximately 30° to the vertical or sagittal plane. This is to keep the needle close to the zygomatic and then the infratemporal surfaces of the maxilla, for if it deviates laterally away from bone it may enter the pterygoid plexus of veins with consequent haematoma formation. The needle also has to pass backwards at an angle of approximately 30° to the occlusal surfaces of the upper teeth.

Because of the lack of bony landmarks it is impossible to be certain when the needle has been inserted to the correct depth other than possibly by radiographic techniques; however, when the marker indicates that it has entered to a depth of 3 cm (*Fig.* 12.9*c*) aspiration is carried out and then 2 ml of solution is slowly injected.

2. GREATER PALATINE APPROACH This consists of the passage of a needle up the greater palatine canal (*Fig.* 12.10*a*), the solution passing out of its superior aspect to reach the maxillary nerve in the region of the infraorbital fissure. The greater palatine nerve and also the descending palatine artery and vein are contained within the relatively narrow confines of the canal and thus some trauma to these structures is bound to

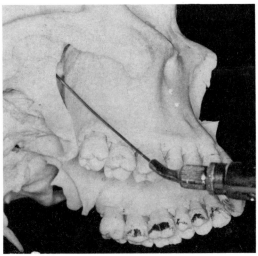

a

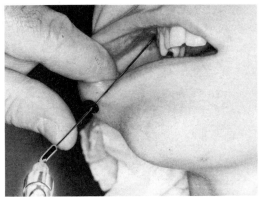

b

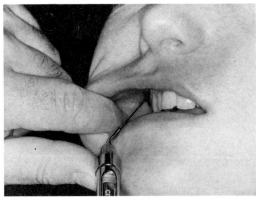

c

Fig. 12.9. *a*, The posterior infraorbital approach to the maxillary nerve. *b*, The site of entry of the needle, which has a marker to indicate the depth of insertion required. *c*, The final position of the needle.

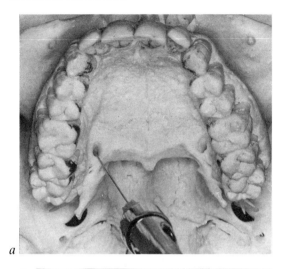

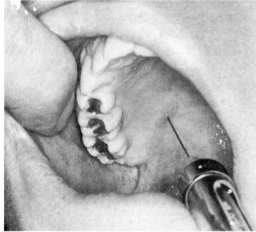

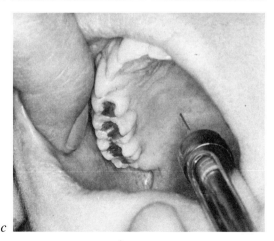

Fig. 12.10. *a*, The greater palatine approach to the maxillary nerve. *b*, The site of entry of the needle. *c*, The final position of the needle.

result when the needle is inserted. Because of the risk of damage to tissues within the canal this type of injection is not recommended, although the injury is likely to be reversible. A fairly rigid needle is required but also one which is not too thick, otherwise it will be unable to pass up the canal.

The foramen is situated at a point half-way between the third molar and the midline. It may be located by a small depression in the overlying mucosa or it may be palpable. The approach is made from the opposite side of the mouth, the needle being gently inserted and a small quantity of solution infiltrated, sufficient time being allowed to elapse for this to take effect. The foramen may now be identified with the needle which enters the canal, passing upwards and backwards at an approximate angle of 45° to the occlusal plane of the upper teeth. It also deviates a little laterally and thus the angulation of the syringe is adjusted to allow for this. The needle should be inserted slowly, altering the angulation as required when bone is felt and avoiding undue force (*Fig.* 12.10*b*). When a depth of 3 cm is achieved aspiration is performed and 2 ml of solution is slowly deposited (*Fig.* 12.10*c*), allowing plenty of time for it to diffuse out through the superior aspect of the canal. On occasions it will be found to be impossible to insert the needle to the correct depth without using excessive force. In these cases one can either abandon the attempt if the needle has been inserted only a little way or, if it is at a depth somewhere approaching that required, inject the solution, as it may diffuse through the canal to reach the maxillary nerve. In these instances analgesia of the posterior superior dental nerve is usually achieved due to the solution diffusing through the relatively porous bone in this region.

A disadvantage of this technique is that it may be painful unless very carefully executed. There is also a greater chance of needle fracture with this injection than any other, as it is held fairly rigidly in the canal and unable to flex; thus, if the patient jerks his head the needle is liable to break at its point of entry and prove difficult to remove.

3. EXTRAORAL APPROACH With any extraoral injection meticulous care should be taken with

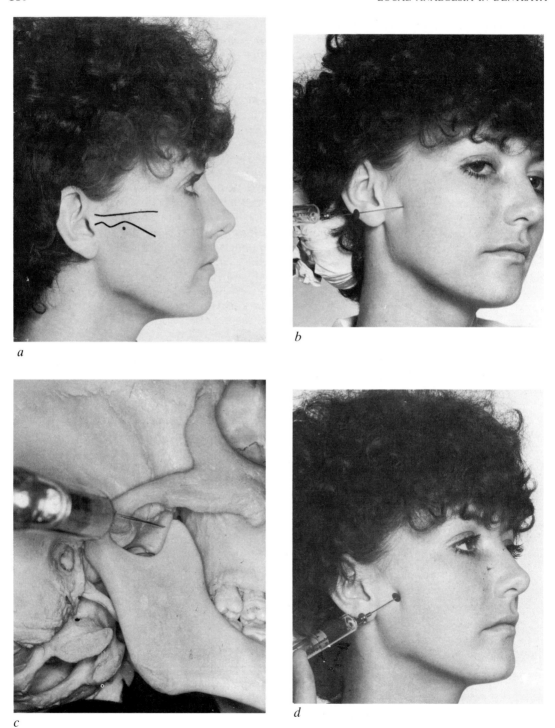

Fig. 12.11. Extraoral maxillary nerve block. *a*, The point of insertion of the needle is below the midpoint of the depression on the lower border of the zygomatic arch. *b*, The site of injection. *c*, The needle is inserted until the lateral pterygoid plate is reached. *d*, The final position of the needle.

cleansing of the site of insertion of the needle because:

a. The pathogenic organisms on the skin are often more virulent than those found in the oral cavity.

b. It is simpler to cleanse the skin than the oral mucosa.

To reach the pterygopalatine fossa from an external approach one has to avoid the coronoid process and thus two techniques are possible: passing the needle either in front of the coronoid or behind it. The latter technique will be described.

The zygomatic process is palpated and the midpoint of the depression on its lower border is marked on the skin (*Fig.* 12.11*a*). Local analgesia is now achieved by infiltration in this area. A heavy-gauge needle of a minimum length of 3 in (75 mm) is used for the injection, incorporating a marker to indicate a depth of 2 in (50 mm), which should never be exceeded.

The needle is inserted at the mark a little below the zygomatic process and at right-angles to the skin surface (*Fig.* 12.11*b*) until the lateral pterygoid plate is reached, thus establishing the depth of insertion required, it normally being less than 5 cm (*Fig.* 12.11*c*). The needle is now largely withdrawn and redirected in a slightly upward (approximately 10°) and slightly forward (approximately 15°) direction when it should pass a little deeper than the initial insertion (*Fig.* 12.11*d*), this being at a maximum of 5 cm if bone has not been previously reached. If it is inserted beyond this, then it may pass into the infraorbital fissure. If the injection has been performed correctly the tip of the needle should be in the pterygopalatine fossa. As this is a highly vascular area, aspiration should always be practised prior to the administration of the local analgesic. If there is a difficulty in manoeuvring the needle past the sigmoid notch then more space will become available by propping the mouth farther open.

Disadvantages of maxillary nerve blocks

1. All techniques for blocking the maxillary nerve involve the passing of a needle into areas of high vascularity with the attendant risk of haemorrhage into the inaccessible deeper tissues.

2. Because of the great depth of insertion of the needle it is extremely difficult to be certain that the correct site has been reached before injecting the analgesic. The complexity of the technique precludes its use where a simpler nerve block would suffice.

3. Should infection result, the consequences, because of the region involved, may be very serious.

4. All the techniques are relatively painful.

5. With the greater palatine approach there is a considerable risk of damage to other anatomical structures in the canal.

6. There is a risk of needle breakage if the greater palatine approach is used.

THE MANDIBULAR NERVE AND ITS BRANCHES

Injections can be used to block the following nerves:

1. The incisive nerve, blocked by the mental injection.
2. The inferior dental nerve.
3. The lingual nerve.
4. The long buccal nerve.
5. The mandibular nerve itself.

1. Mental and incisive nerves

The term *mental injection* is a somewhat confusing one, as its main purpose is to block not the mental nerve but the incisive nerve, which

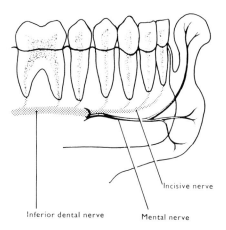

*Fig.*12.12. The mental and incisive nerves.

is the terminal branch of the inferior dental. The mental nerve emerges from its foramen to innervate the mucosa and skin of the lower lip and chin and the buccal and labial gingivae associated with the first premolar, canine and incisor teeth, and is also affected by this injection. The incisive nerve supplies the pulps, alveolar process and periodontal membrane of the lower incisors, canine and first premolar (*Fig.* 12.12).

The injection derives its name from the fact that it makes use of the mental foramen to allow analgesic solution to enter the inferior dental canal. As well as the teeth supplied by the incisive nerve, the second premolar is also usually affected as the solution diffuses back down the inferior dental canal.

Techniques

This nerve is usually blocked by an intraoral approach, although very rarely an extraoral

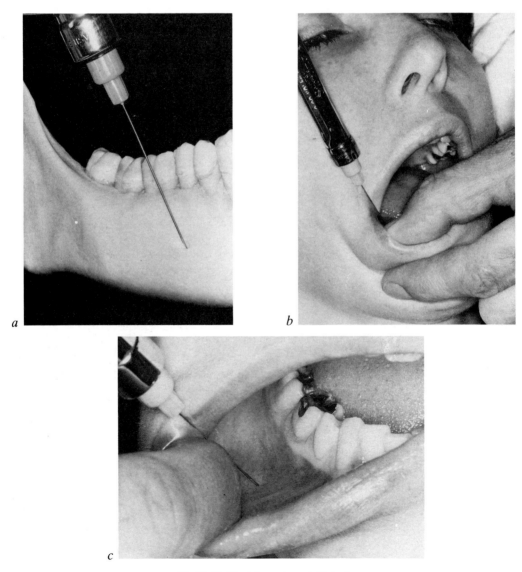

Fig. 12.13. The intraoral mental injection.

approach may be used when access to the oral cavity is difficult or infection of the mucosa is present.

1. INTRAORAL APPROACH The mental foramen usually lies below the apex of the second premolar or, less commonly, below and between the apices of the lower first and second premolars. However, its position is variable and thus if a radiograph is available it is useful to note the site of the mental foramen relative to the premolars. It faces posteriorly and thus when making an injection the approach should be from behind. The lip and cheek are retracted to allow insertion of the syringe fitted with a 27-gauge $1\frac{5}{8}$-in (42-mm) needle from as far back as possible, the mouth being partly closed to relax the oral musculature and save the patient discomfort (*Fig.* 12.13). The mental foramen is palpated and the finger left there, the needle being inserted a little behind the second premolar and passed downwards and a little forwards for approximately 1 cm. A few drops of analgesic are then deposited and if this is at the mental foramen the solution will be felt by the finger distending the tissues. Approximately 1·5 ml of solution are slowly injected and gentle massage is employed to stimulate the flow of the solution into the canal.

In the elderly, particularly the edentulous, the mental foramen assumes a position far nearer the crest of the lower ridge (*Fig.* 12.14) and indeed, on occasions, pressure intraorally, near the crest of the ridge in the mental region, will produce pain in the lower lip, indicating the extremely superficial position of the nerve.

2. EXTRAORAL APPROACH The mandible is palpated externally in the region below the apex of the second premolar, where a depression indicating the presence of the mental foramen can be felt. This normally lies equidistant between the upper and lower borders of the mandible when teeth are present.

The skin is carefully cleaned with an antiseptic such as chlorhexidine gluconate and a 25-gauge 1-in (2·5 cm) needle is passed downwards at an angle of 30° and forwards at an angle of 45° to the body of the mandible until bone is reached; the angle of insertion of the needle thus corresponds with the angle of the mental foramen. A small quantity of analgesic is then injected and some 15–20 seconds allowed to elapse for this to take effect. The foramen is now located with the needle, which is then gently inserted for a short distance, and approximately 1 ml of solution is slowly injected. The needle is removed and massage carried out to aid the diffusion of the solution into the mental foramen and along the incisive and inferior dental canals.

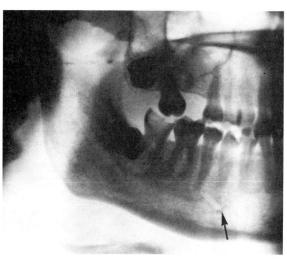

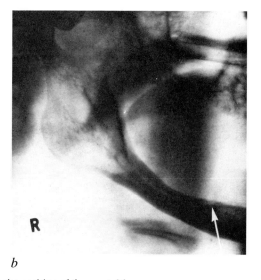

a   *b*

Fig. 12.14. Radiographs showing variations in the position of the mental foramen.

Advantages

A mental injection avoids the unpleasant loss of
lingual sensation which generally occurs with an
inferior dental injection. This is especially
important with children, who are liable to bite
their tongues.

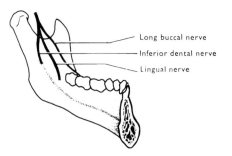

Fig. 12.16. Lingual view of mandible with shaded line
indicating the inferior dental canal.

Complications and contraindications

Complications with these injections are rare,
although failures are occasionally experienced
because of the small size of the mental foramen
through which the solution reaches the canal. In
these instances it is best to resort to an inferior
dental nerve block.

It should be remembered that the lower
central incisors and, to a lesser degree, the
lateral incisors derive some innervation from
the incisive nerve of the opposite side, therefore, analgesia of these teeth will not be
achieved with a single mental nerve block.
Where analgesia of only these teeth is required
a supraperiosteal injection should be used.

2. The inferior dental nerve

The inferior dental nerve block is by far the
commonest used in dentistry, the reason being
that it is a very satisfactory way of achieving
analgesia of the lower molars. However, for the
premolars one has the choice of either a mental

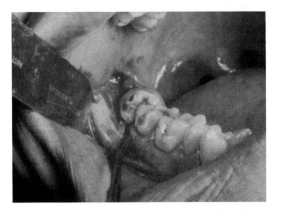

Fig. 12.15. In the lower molar region the buccal bone,
seen here during removal of a third molar, is too thick for
infiltration analgesia.

or an inferior dental nerve block. An infiltration
technique is almost invariably unsuccessful in
the molar region because of the thickness and
density of the buccal alveolar bone (*Fig*. 12.15),
and even in the premolar region the bone is
comparatively thick. Intraligamentary injections may be used to obtain analgesia of
individual teeth. The lingual nerve is generally
affected at the same time when an inferior
dental injection is given, as the two nerves are in
fairly close proximity (*Fig*. 12.16). The usual
exception to the use of the inferior dental nerve
block is where conservation of the lower premolars, canine or incisors is to be performed
and analgesia of the lingual aspects of these
teeth is not normally required. Here one may
use a mental injection and thus avoid analgesia
of the tongue. An infiltration injection is usually
adequate for the lower canine or incisors. The
dangers inherent in administering block
injections, particularly the inferior dental, to
patients suffering from haemorrhagic diatheses
such as haemophilia have been noted in
Chapter 7. Experimental jet injection blocks
have been mentioned in Chapter 10.

At one time it was considered unsafe to
administer bilateral inferior dental blocks on
the same occasion because of the risk of the
patient losing control of the tongue, it being
thought that proprioceptive innervation of the
tongue was via the lingual nerves. However,
Adatia and Gehring (1972) carried out a careful
clinical trial to research this problem and concluded that bilateral inferior dental and lingual
nerve blocks were well tolerated by patients.
All their patients retained full control of the
lingual musculature and positional sense of
the tongue.

Technique: general considerations

The inferior dental nerve is blocked by the deposition of analgesic solution around it just before it enters the mandibular foramen and when it is in the pterygomandibular space. This is bounded laterally by the ascending ramus and medially by the medial pterygoid muscle, the posterior boundary being the parotid gland containing branches of the facial nerve (*Fig. 12.17*).

There are many techniques for the administration of an inferior dental nerve block, but the two main ones are the 'direct' and 'indirect' methods, and of these, the direct technique is usually preferable. The direct technique is recommended, but if the operator considers that the syringe needle has contacted bone at too shallow a depth of needle insertion then the injection should proceed as described for the indirect method.

Before proceeding with the injection, it is important to assess each case carefully as there can be a considerable variation in the position of the mandibular foramen relative to the landmarks used when an injection is given.

FACTORS AFFECTING THE RELATIVE POSITION OF THE MANDIBULAR FORAMEN

a. Width of ascending ramus: The greater the width of the ascending ramus, then the farther

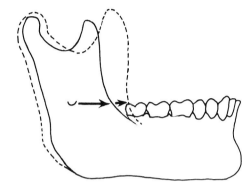

Fig. 12.18. The relative position of the mandibular foramen will vary with the width of the ascending ramus as shown by the arrow.

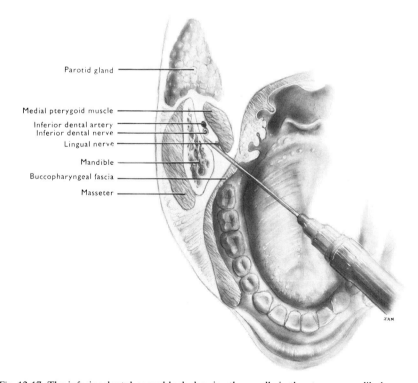

Parotid gland

Medial pterygoid muscle
Inferior dental artery
Inferior dental nerve
Lingual nerve
Mandible
Buccopharyngeal fascia
Masseter

Fig. 12.17. The inferior dental nerve block showing the needle in the pterygomandibular space.

back the mandibular foramen will be situated and thus the deeper the needle will have to be inserted (*Fig.* 12.18).

b. Width of arch of the mandible: The wider the arch then the farther back the body of the syringe will have to be placed on the opposite side to the injection in order to allow the needle to clear the internal oblique ridge and still reach the mandibular foramen (*Fig.* 12.19).

c. Obliquity of the angle of the mandible: The more oblique the angle of the mandible then the farther forward and the higher up the mandibular foramen will be and thus the injection technique will need to be modified accordingly (*Fig.* 12.20).

Direct technique

The method for administering a right inferior dental nerve block, assuming that the operator is right-handed, is described below.

The operator stands (or sits) in front of the patient, who is positioned comfortably. A syringe with a $1\frac{5}{8}$-in (42-mm) needle of 26 gauge is used. A short needle should be avoided because of the increased risk of breakage which occurs when a needle is inserted into the tissues up to the hub.

To locate the point of insertion of the needle the index finger of the left hand is moved distally in the mucobuccal fold until the external oblique ridge is felt at the anterior aspect of the ascending ramus (*Fig.* 12.21). The finger is now rotated so that the nail faces lingually and then the retromolar triangle or fossa is palpated (*Fig.* 12.22*a*), this being bounded medially by the internal oblique ridge to which the pterygomandibular raphe is attached. The needle is inserted from the left side of the mouth, the barrel of the syringe lying midway between the left lower premolars. The needle enters the tissues at a point bisecting the fingernail of

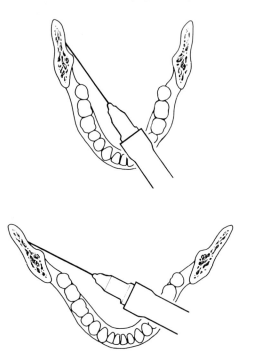

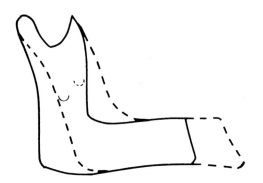

Fig. 12.19. The correct position of the syringe will vary with the width of the arch of the mandible.

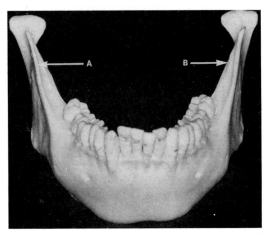

Fig. 12.20. The more oblique the angle of the mandible the higher up and farther forward is the mandibular foramen.

Fig. 12.21. The mandible, showing landmarks for the inferior dental injection. A, External oblique ridge. B, Internal oblique ridge.

the guide finger and about 0·5 cm medially to it, passing into the tissues between the pterygomandibular raphe and the mandible (*Fig.* 12.22*b*). The needle is slowly inserted to a depth of approximately 1 cm and if lingual analgesia is required then 0·5 ml of solution is injected at this point. The needle is now passed deeper into the tissues until bone is contacted and then withdrawn 1 mm prior to aspiration and then the remainder of the solution is slowly deposited (*Fig.* 12.22*c*). The total depth of insertion is usually 2–2·5 cm, but this may be modified because of the anatomical variations mentioned earlier. To minimize discomfort a little solution should be infiltrated during the

passage of the needle to achieve analgesia of the deeper tissues before the needle penetrates them.

CORRECTIONS FOR ANATOMICAL VARIATIONS

a. If bone is struck soon after insertion, that is with only about 5 mm of needle inserted, then the needle must be withdrawn a little and the body of the syringe swung over to a line parallel with the right lower molars so as to disengage the needle from bone (*Fig.* 12.22*d*). This modification makes the technique similar to the indirect method, which is described later. The needle is then inserted deeper for approximately 7 mm prior to swinging the syringe back

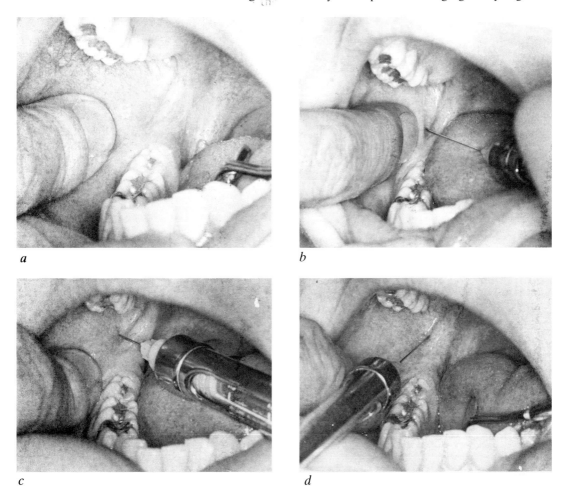

a

b

c

d

Fig. 12.22. Inferior dental nerve block. *a*, The index finger palpates the external oblique ridge. *b*, The needle enters the tissues at a point bisecting the fingernail. *c*, The index finger has been moved to show the final position of the needle. *d*, If bone is struck too soon after insertion the needle is partially withdrawn and its direction corrected to avoid the internal oblique ridge.

to its original direction, when the needle is then inserted to the correct depth which is reached when the point touches bone again.

  b. If bone is not reached after insertion of the needle for a reasonable distance, that is up to 3 cm, then an injection should not be made on the assumption that the point of the needle is near the inferior dental foramen. It is more likely to be in the parotid gland, and thus not far from the facial nerve, or too far medially, and therefore in the medial pterygoid muscle. The needle should be almost completely withdrawn, the barrel of the syringe swung farther back on the left side, and the needle reinserted until its point touches bone.

LEFT INFERIOR DENTAL NERVE BLOCK To administer a left inferior dental nerve block it is desirable to reverse the role of the hands and use the left hand to hold the syringe. In this way one can again stand (or sit) in front of the patient, which greatly facilitates the estimation of the point of insertion of the needle and the angle of the syringe. Most operators can rapidly acquire sufficient dexterity with their left hand to carry out this simple procedure but, if it is beyond their capabilities, then the injection may be a modification of that described for the right inferior dental nerve block and administered from behind the patient. Then the right hand is used for holding the syringe and the left arm passed around behind the patient's head, the retromolar region being palpated with the left forefinger to locate the site for insertion of the needle.

Alternative techniques

1. THE INDIRECT METHOD The technique for a right inferior dental nerve block is described (*Fig.* 12.23), a relatively rigid needle being required with a minimum gauge of 25. With the indirect technique the midline of the fingernail again indicates the point of insertion of the needle, this being 1 cm above the occlusal plane of the lower teeth. However, the finger is placed on the external oblique ridge, as opposed to the retromolar fossa with the direct method. Thus, the initial insertion of the needle is more lateral and it almost immediately strikes bone (*Fig.* 12.24*a,b*). The barrel of the syringe is now

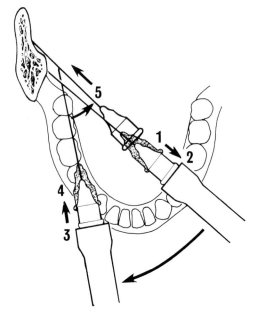

Fig. 12.23. Stages in the indirect technique for the inferior dental nerve block. 1, (shaded) initial insertion of the needle. 2, Its partial withdrawal after touching bone. 3, The syringe is moved parallel to the lower molars on the other side. 4, (Shaded) the insertion of the needle point beyond the internal oblique ridge. 5, The syringe is returned to its original direction and the injection is completed.

moved to the right until it is parallel with the right lower molars (*Fig.* 12.24*c, d*). A few drops of analgesic solution are deposited and about 10 seconds allowed to elapse prior to inserting the needle approximately 7 mm, thus passing it on the medial aspect of the internal oblique ridge. The syringe is now swung back to the left side of the mouth, the barrel being replaced over the lower premolars. The needle is gently inserted until it reaches the pterygomandibular space and strikes bone; it is then withdrawn a little to avoid injecting subperiosteally, prior to slowly depositing approximately 1·5 ml of the solution (*Fig.* 12.24*e, f*). If it is required to block the lingual nerve, as for extractions, then the remainder of the solution is injected after the syringe has been withdrawn half-way. However, even without this addition to the technique, the lingual nerve is often affected.

  Where satisfactory analgesia is not obtained by either the direct or indirect methods already described, then recourse may be made to other techniques.

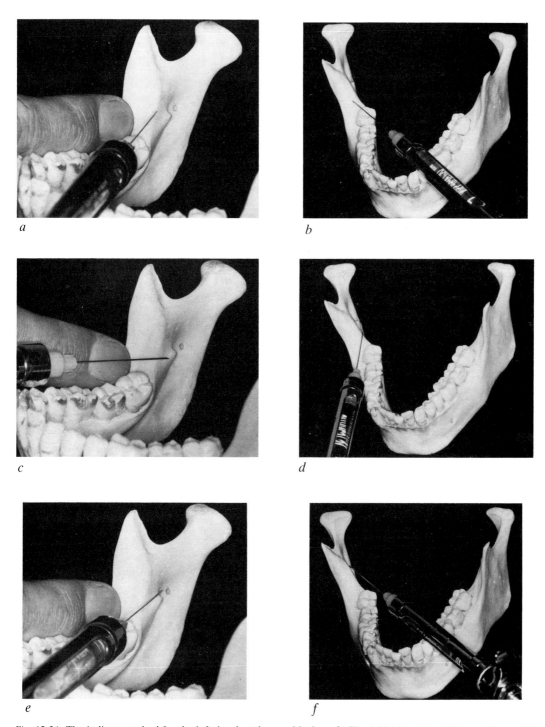

Fig. 12.24. The indirect method for the inferior dental nerve block. *a*, *b*, The initial insertion of the needle. *c*, *d*, The syringe is moved parallel to the lower molars. *e*, *f*, The final position of the needle.

2. METHOD OF CLARKE AND HOLMES (1959) This involves the deposition of the solution at a higher level than usual. The reasoning behind this is that when the standard direct or indirect technique is employed the analgesic is placed immediately behind the mandibular foramen which is approximately 1 cm above the occlusal plane of the molar teeth. At this level the anterior part of the nerve is concealed by the lingula and the sphenomandibular ligament and so local analgesic solution may have some difficulty in diffusing to the well-protected anterior fibres. It is also likely that branches are sometimes given off from the inferior dental nerve a little before it reaches the inferior dental foramen, these fibres entering the bone by separate foramina around and above the main one. By depositing the solution at a higher level it reaches the nerve in a position where it is not protected and before it has given off any branches.

This technique is a modification of the indirect method. The patient is instructed to keep the mouth wide open and the head-rest is adjusted so that the lower occlusal plane is parallel to the floor. Assuming that a right inferior dental nerve block is to be administered, the index finger is slid along the occlusal surfaces of the molar teeth and the external oblique ridge is palpated. The finger is then rotated inwards so that the tip lies in the retromolar fossa and the fingernail overlies the internal oblique ridge.

A syringe equipped with a long needle is used, it being advanced from between the premolars on the opposite side, the point passing into the tissue just above the fingernail of the index finger (*Fig.* 12.25*a*) and not at the midpoint as with the standard indirect technique. The needle is inserted for a short distance until bone is encountered. The body of the syringe is then gently swung round until it lies over the lower central incisors, keeping it parallel to the molar teeth in a horizontal plane at the same time. The needle is passed another 2 cm deeper into the tissues and after this 1·5 ml of solution are slowly deposited (*Fig.* 12.25*b,c*). At this point the analgesic will have been injected more than 1 cm higher than usual.

Should lingual analgesia be required then the remainder of the solution is deposited when the needle is being withdrawn.

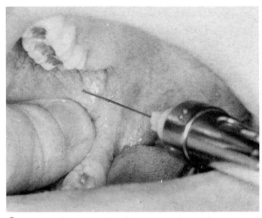

a

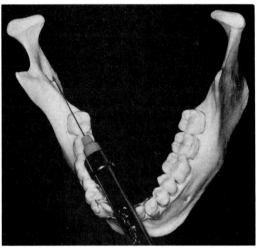

b

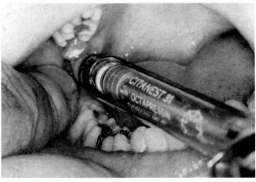

c

Fig. 12.25. The technique of Clarke and Holmes for regional analgesia of the inferior dental nerve. The needle is inserted at a higher level than that used in the indirect technique. In the final position the barrel of the syringe is lying over the central incisors.

3. METHOD OF ANGELO SARGENTI (1966) The technique employed by Sargenti for achieving analgesia of the inferior dental nerve is a modification of the direct method already described. The principal difference is that the nerve is approached from a higher level than usual.

A syringe with a $1\frac{5}{8}$-in (42-mm) 26-gauge needle is used. The index finger is placed in the retromolar fossa with the nail facing lingually. The point of the needle is then inserted opposite the midpoint of the fingernail and a little

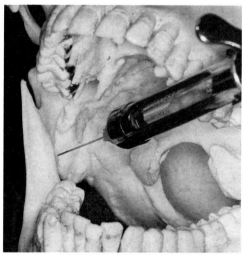

a

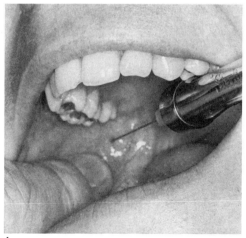

b

Fig. 12.26. Regional analgesia of the inferior dental nerve using the technique of Angelo Sargenti. The barrel of the syringe is kept in contact with the upper premolar teeth.

beyond its tip. The barrel of the syringe is now placed between and in contact with the upper premolars of the opposite side and it is kept in this position while the needle is slowly inserted in a downwards and backwards direction until it touches bone, which is usually at a depth of 1 cm. For this injection 1·5 ml of analgesic solution will usually suffice (*Fig.* 12.26).

4. METHOD OF SUNDER J. VAZIRANI (1960) Where the patient is unable to open his mouth then the technique described by S. J. Vazirani may be used (*Fig.* 12.27*a,b*). The only contra-indication is where trismus is due to infection in the tissues through which a needle would have to pass.

With the patient's mouth closed, the cheek is retracted laterally, and the syringe, equipped with a long needle, inserted in such a way that the needle is placed parallel to the gingival margins of the maxillary teeth or to the alveolar ridge in the edentulous patient. The point of insertion is the pterygomandibular fold, the needle passing through the mucosa, buccinator and buccal aponeurosis on the inner aspect of the ascending ramus to reach the pterygo-mandibular space, where the solution is slowly deposited (*Fig.* 12.27*c*). The total depth of insertion of the needle is usually about 1·5 cm.

The onset of analgesia with this method is somewhat slower than with the direct technique and it is desirable to use a larger quantity of analgesic.

5. EXTERNAL APPROACH This technique is only used when there is severe limitation of opening of the jaws, for example, as may occur with ankylosis of the temporomandibular joints. Because the injection is an external one, great care must be taken with cleansing of the skin prior to injection to reduce the risk of infecting the deeper tissues.

This method has been attributed to Professor Kurt Thoma. First, the anterior border of the masseter is located by getting the patient to clench the teeth. The operator's finger is then run down this border until its lowest point is found. This point is marked and a line drawn connecting this with the tragus of the ear. The midpoint of this line is noted as it marks externally the position of the mandibular foramen

(*Fig.* 12.28). A line is drawn down from this point parallel with the posterior border of the mandible to the lower border. This line is now measured and a 21-gauge needle of 7–8 cm

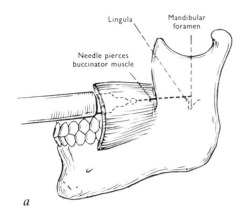

a

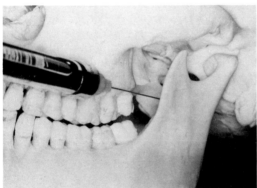

b

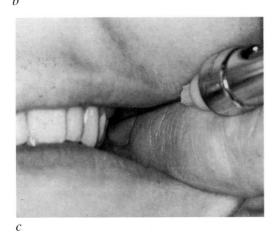

c

Fig. 12.27. Regional analgesia of the inferior dental nerve using the closed-mouth technique of Sunder J. Vazirani. (*Fig.* 12.27*a* reproduced from S. J. Vazirani (1960) *Dent. Dig.* **66,** 10).

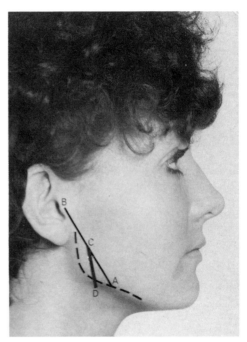

Fig. 12.28. Surface markings used for assessing the position of the mandibular foramen. A, Lowest point on the anterior border of the masseter. B, Tragus. C, Midpoint of line AB. Line CD is parallel to the posterior border of the ascending ramus. D, Point of insertion of needle.

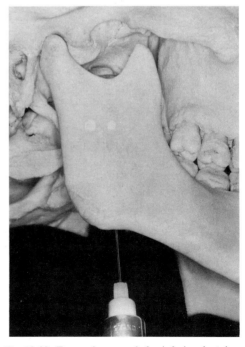

Fig. 12.29. External approach for inferior dental nerve block. Skull, showing position of the needle.

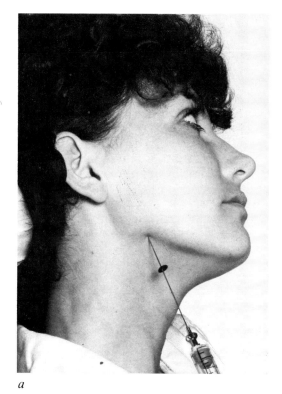

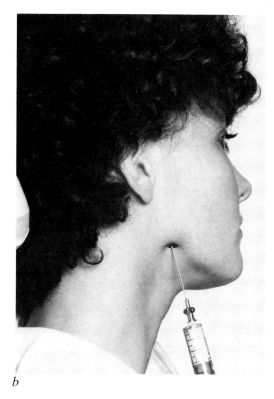

a   b

Fig. 12.30. *a,* Point of entry of needle. A marker has been placed on it to show correct depth of insertion. *b,* Needle in its final position with the marker touching the skin.

length is marked to a similar length by means of a piece of rubber dam or other suitable method.

After cleansing the skin, an infiltration injection is made in the area with a fine-gauge needle to obtain local analgesia. The long needle is now inserted on the inner aspect of the lower border of the mandible, care being taken to keep it as near bone as possible throughout the injection (*Fig.* 12.29).

The needle is gradually inserted, taking great care to keep it parallel with the line marked on the skin of the external surface of the mandible. When it has reached the depth indicated by the marker, that is opposite the point marked on the skin overlying the position of the foramen, the solution is slowly injected (*Fig.* 12.30).

3. The lingual nerve

This passes down deep to the lateral pterygoid until its lower border is reached, at which point it lies anterior to the inferior dental nerve (*Fig.*

12.31). It then runs downwards and forwards to a position on the lingual side of the third molar just above the posterior end of the mylohyoid line and it is here that its conduction can be conveniently blocked. After this it continues downwards and forwards and then divides, some fibres going to the mucous membrane of the floor of the mouth and the lingual aspect of the lower teeth and others supplying the anterior two-thirds of the tongue (*Fig.* 9.1).

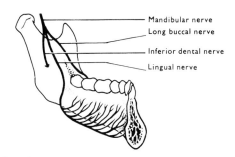

Fig. 12.31. The inner aspect of the mandible showing the lingual nerve.

Analgesia may be achieved by three methods:

1. Blocking the lingual nerve at the same time as an intraoral inferior dental injection is administered by the deposition of 0·5 ml of solution after the needle has been inserted for approximately 1 cm and before it has reached the inferior dental nerve (*Fig.* 12.17).

2. The submucosal infiltration of 0·5 ml of analgesic a few millimetres below and behind the region of the lower third molar on its lingual aspect (*Fig.* 12.32).

3. The infiltration of analgesic solution immediately lingual to the gingivae or mucosa to be treated (*Fig.* 12.33).

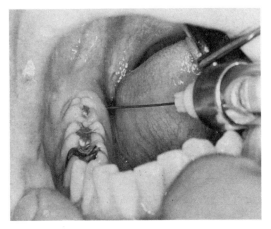

Fig. 12.32. Analgesia of the lingual nerve may be obtained by submucosal infiltration below and behind the third molar region.

4. The long buccal nerve

This is a branch of the anterior division of the mandibular nerve. It passes downwards between the two heads of the lateral pterygoid to reach the anterior border of the masseter behind and at a similar occlusal level to the lower third molar. It then divides, some fibres passing medially to pierce the buccinator and supply the buccal gingivae of the lower posterior region and the adjoining mucous membrane, and other fibres continuing forwards to innervate the skin of the cheek (*Fig.* 12.34).

Analgesia of the long buccal as well as the inferior dental and lingual nerves is always required when extracting mandibular molars. In a considerable proportion of cases this will be achieved without recourse to a separate injection when an inferior dental nerve block is administered, but to be certain of analgesia an injection should be given into the buccal mucosa immediately distal to the region it is required to treat as the terminal branches of the nerve run forwards beneath the mucosa lining the buccal sulcus. Alternatively, one may inject submucosally at the point where the nerve crosses the external oblique ridge on the distobuccal aspect of the lower third molar (*Fig.* 12.35). Whichever technique is used, only about 0·5 ml of solution need be injected, and the former technique is recommended as it is more reliable.

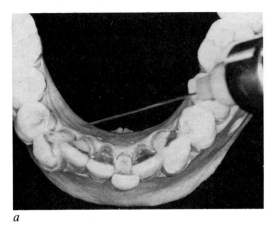

a

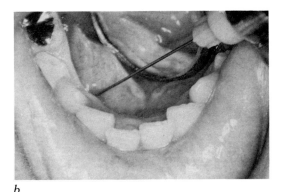

b

Fig. 12.33. Lingual infiltration in the region of the lower canine. The mouth mirror is used to retract the tongue and also to reflect light on to the site of injection.

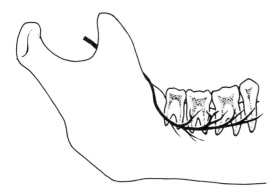

Fig. 12.34. The outer aspect of the mandible showing the long buccal nerve.

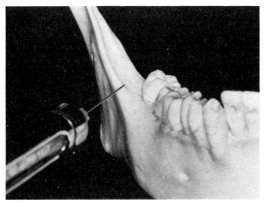

a

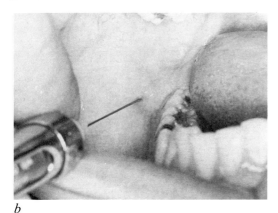

b

Fig. 12.35. Analgesia of the long buccal nerve by injection near the external oblique ridge.

5. The mandibular nerve

The entire mandibular branch of the trigeminal nerve may be blocked. This injection should not be confused with the inferior dental nerve block which is sometimes erroneously referred to as a 'mandibular'.

Uses

This nerve block is of particular use in the diagnosis of facial pains such as causalgias and *tic douloureux*. If the pain seems to affect the mandibular nerve then this injection may be tried to see if it relieves the pain before a trigeminal block is attempted. It is often advisable to try an inferior dental nerve block in the first instance to check if this eliminates or produces any alleviation of symptoms.

Techniques

1. INTRAORAL GOW-GATES' METHOD (1973) Using a 5-ml aspirating syringe with a long needle, the mucosa in the buccal sulcus opposite the maxillary third molar is penetrated, the mucosa being distended so that the deep fibres and tendon of temporalis are compressed laterally against the anterior border of the vertical ramus of the mandible, the patient's mouth being widely open. The point of insertion of the needle is a higher puncture point than for the inferior dental nerve block, very close but medial to the temporalis, and lateral to the pterygotemporal depression. At this stage the needle is parallel to a plane joining the corner of the mouth and the apex of the intertragic notch of the external ear (*Fig*. 12.36). The syringe may be held in a pen grip and directed towards the posterior border of the tragus to contact the condylar neck with the needle inserted to a depth of about 25–27 mm. The needle is aimed much more laterally than with an inferior dental nerve block, and if the condylar neck is not contacted at a depth of about 27 mm then the approach should be reassessed. The syringe usually lies above the incisal edge of the canine of the opposite side but there is wide variation. If the syringe is angled too far laterally then the point of the needle may have entered the sigmoid notch. After contacting the condylar neck, the syringe is withdrawn about a millimetre (*Fig*. 12.37), aspirated to check that an intravascular injection is not given, and about 3 ml of local anaesthetic solution slowly injected. With this technique, having the mouth widely

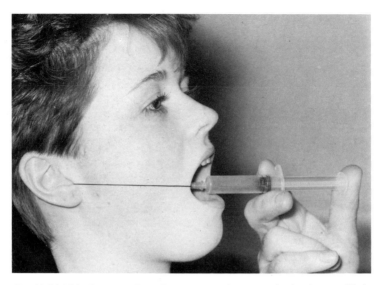

Fig. 12.36. This shows the Gow-Gates' approach to anaesthetize the mandibular nerve. The line on the face shows the syringe is directed towards the intertragic notch of the ear.

open brings the condylar neck and the mandibular nerve into a more anterior position. For this reason the mouth should still be kept open for about half a minute while the local anaesthetic solution bathes the nerve.

This injection should numb completely the mandibular nerve so that there is analgesia in the distribution of the inferior dental, lingual, long buccal and associated nerves. Levy (1981) assessed the Gow-Gates' injection and compared it with the inferior dental nerve block on a series of 26 patients requiring bilateral removal of mandibular third molars. He reported complete analgesia for about 96 per cent of the Gow-Gates' injections compared with 65 per cent for the inferior dental nerve blocks. Patients thought that onset of analgesia was somewhat slower with the Gow-

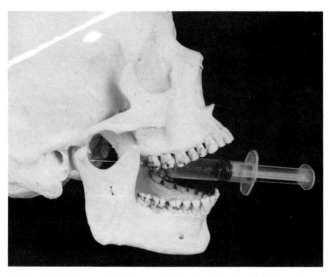

Fig. 12.37. The point of the needle is situated a short distance from the condylar neck prior to injecting.

Gates' technique, and occasionally the long buccal and auriculotemporal nerves were not anaesthetized.

2. EXTRAORAL APPROACH This injection is very similar to the maxillary nerve block, the two nerves being in quite close apposition immediately after they leave the skull, the maxillary nerve through the foramen rotundum and the mandibular nerve via the adjacent foramen ovale. The aim of the technique is to achieve analgesia of the nerve just after it emerges from the foramen (*Fig.* 12.38).

The point of maximum concavity in the lower border of the zygomatic process is located by palpation and this point marked on the skin (*Fig.* 12.39). This area should be cleansed and then local analgesia obtained with an infiltration injection using a fine needle.

A 21-gauge $3\frac{1}{8}$-in (8-cm) needle, marked to a depth of 4 cm, is now inserted at right-angles to the sagittal or vertical axis of the patient and also at right angles to the skin (*Fig.* 12.40*a*). The

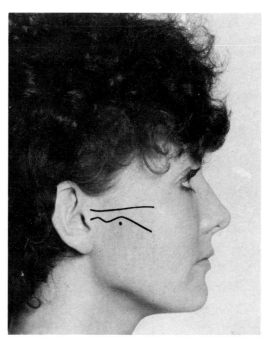

Fig. 12.39. The surface markings for the external mandibular nerve block. The point of insertion of the needle is below the midpoint of the depression on the lower border of the zygomatic arch.

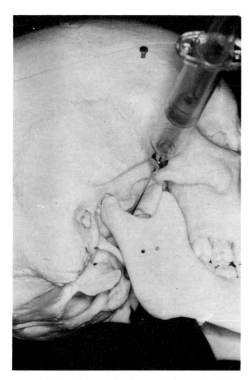

Fig. 12.38. Infralateral view of skull showing the needle is below the midpoint of the depression on the lower border of the zygomatic arch.

needle is slowly inserted until the lateral pterygoid plate is reached, which should be at a depth of approximately 4 cm. The needle is now withdrawn and reinserted a few degrees farther distally so as to pass just behind the posterior border of the lateral pterygoid plate. If this is achieved, it will be possible to insert the needle to a greater depth. However, the needle should not be inserted more than 4 mm beyond the established depth of the lateral pterygoid plate and on no account to more than a total depth of 5 cm (*Fig.* 12.40*b*). Now 2 ml of the solution is injected and this should produce analgesia of the mandibular teeth, the side of tongue, the lower lip, the skin of the cheek innervated by the long buccal nerve and the skin overlying the temple.

An unusual complication of an extraoral injection to block the right maxillary and mandibular branches of the trigeminal nerve was reported by Nique and Bennett (1981). An injection of 5 ml of 0·25 per cent bupivacaine hydrochloride had been given via the extraoral lateral pterygoid plate approach using an aspirating technique, and within 60 seconds the patient's voice became hoarse, the right pupil dilated and 2 minutes or so later she became unconscious with respiratory arrest and bilaterally dilated pupils. She was intubated,

given positive-pressure ventilation with oxygen, and subsequently recovered due to the prompt resuscitative measures. It was considered that the cause of the inadvertent brainstem anaesthesia was due to bupivacaine being injected directly into the subarachnoid space with the needle entering the foramen ovale or penetrating the dural sleeve which anatomically may be below the level of the cranial base. It is possible that the needle was inserted too deeply when this extraoral block was administered, but of primary importance is the swift recognition of the complication and administration of effective emergency treatment.

CAUSES OF FAILURE OF REGIONAL ANALGESIA

Most of the factors responsible for an infiltration injection failing to achieve analgesia also apply to a regional nerve block; however, the

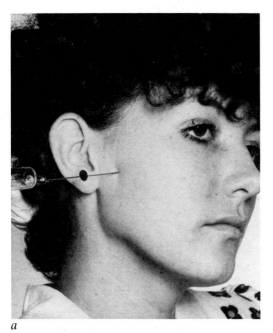

a

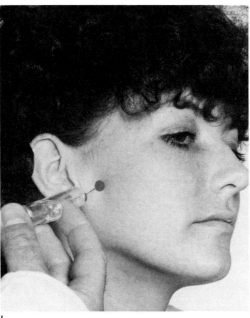

b

Fig. 12.40. External mandibular nerve block. *a*, The initial insertion of the needle. *b*, The final position of the needle.

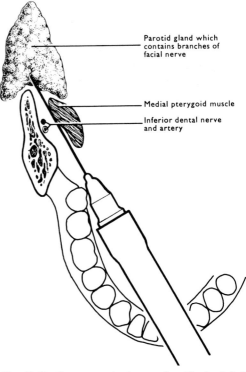

Parotid gland which contains branches of facial nerve

Medial pterygoid muscle

Inferior dental nerve and artery

Fig. 12.41. Common mistakes made with the inferior dental injection. The angulation of the syringe is wrong because its barrel is overlying the incisors and not the premolars. Thus the needle has passed too far medially, missing the ascending ramus. The needle has then been inserted too deeply, and has entered the parotid.

most important factor is the deposition of the solution in the wrong site which may be due to several causes:

1. Insufficient knowledge of the local anatomy of the region.

2. Individual anatomical variations occuring in different patients, especially those factors affecting the relative position of the mandibular foramen mentioned earlier in this chapter.

3. Variations due to age:

a. In children the mandibular foramen is relatively lower than in adults.

b. In the edentulous adult reduction in depth of the body of the mandible occurs due to resorption of alveolar bone. Care should be taken to avoid inserting the needle at too low a level in these patients when administering an inferior dental nerve block.

4. Faulty technique. Some of the complications described in Chapter 14 are the results of faulty technique. With the inferior dental nerve block the commonest errors are:

a. Injecting too far posteriorly because the barrel of the syringe is not far enough back over the opposite premolars (*Fig.* 12.41).

b. Injecting too low down. This is often because the lower lip is allowed to lie between the barrel of the syringe and the teeth, thus giving it a downward angulation.

REFERENCES AND FURTHER READING

Adatia A. K. (1968) Posterior superior alveolar nerve block. *Dent. Practit.* **18**, 321.

Adatia A. K. (1976) Regional nerve block for maxillary permanent molars. *Br. Dent. J.* **140**, 87.

Adatia A. K. and Gehring E. N. (1972) Bilateral inferior alveolar and lingual nerve blocks. *Br. Dent. J.* **133**, 377.

Clarke J. and Holmes G. (1959) Local anaesthesia of the mandibular molar teeth—a new technique. *Dent. Practnr. Dent. Rec.* **10**, 36.

Gow-Gates G. A. E. (1973) Mandibular conduction anesthesia: a new technique using extraoral landmarks. *Oral Surg.* **36**, 321.

Levy T. P. (1981) An assessment of the Gow-Gates mandibular block for third molar surgery. *J. Am. Dent. Assoc.* **103**, 37.

Nique T. A. and Bennett C. R. (1981) Inadvertent brainstem anaesthesia following extraoral trigeminal V2–V3 blocks. *Oral Surg.* **51**, 468.

Petersen J. K. (1971) The mandibular foramen block. *Br. J. Oral Surg.* **9**, 126.

Sargenti A. (1966) *Local Anaesthesia in Dentistry* (Trans. Moore J. R.). London, Kimpton.

Thoma K. H. (1963) *Oral Surgery*, 4th ed., vol. 1. St Louis, Mosby, pp. 152–158.

Vazirani S. J. (1960) Closed mouth mandibular nerve block—a new technique. *Dent. Dig.* **66**, 10.

Chapter 13

SEDATION TECHNIQUES

PREMEDICATION

Premedication is the use of drugs to sedate a patient prior to operative treatment. When used before the administration of a local analgesic, the aim is to make the patient less aware of any discomfort and thus more relaxed and co-operative. When premedication is used prior to treatment under general anaesthesia, and also occasionally when local analgesia is employed, an antisialogogue such as atropine is included. This reduces mucous and serous secretions and thus helps to keep the mouth dry during treatment.

Premedication is more difficult to arrange for patients receiving local analgesia than for those having general anaesthesia (*Fig.* 13.1). This is because it does not matter if the premedication of a patient receiving a general anaesthetic induces sleep prior to its administration and also because this patient is not usually an outpatient who has to return home soon after treatment. For this reason one tends to give people having local analgesia either very mild sedation or no drugs at all. This latter choice is not to be totally disregarded because one study showed that a reassuring talk with the anaesthetist produced a greater calming effect than a premedicant. Unfortunately this soothing manner is not the possession of all operators.

The assessment of the correct dosage for oral premedication of an outpatient is extremely difficult because there is a great individual variation in response to these drugs. Indeed, even in the same person the response may vary widely because of factors such as whether the patient is feeling more apprehensive than usual, whether he is fatigued, and even whether he has recently eaten.

When premedicating a child, it does not usually matter so much if they become a little drowsy as normally they will be accompanied by a responsible person. Dosages obtained by Clarke's rule, where

$$dosage = \frac{weight\ in\ lb \times adult\ dose}{150}$$

or Young's rule, where

$$dosage = \frac{age \times adult\ dose}{age + 12}$$

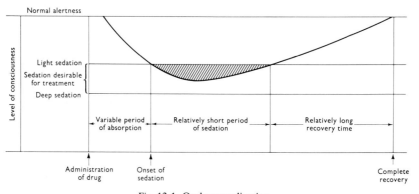

Fig. 13.1. Oral premedication.

130

may prove to be inadequate for achieving pre-medication which will reduce anxiety and encourage the child to accept routine dental treatment calmly. This is primarily because a child has a higher metabolic rate than an adult.

For work under local analgesia, premedication administered orally is usually preferred by the patient, because it is sometimes the thought of an injection that is causing the patient apprehension. Well-tried drugs which are suitable include diazepam, morphine and morphine derivatives such as pethidine (Meperidine, USP). Unfortunately, the wide general use of barbiturates has led to problems of drug dependence and thus their use is best avoided.

Occasionally it is an advantage for the operator to reduce the patient's salivation and then atropine or promethazine may be given about 1–2 hours preoperatively to produce inhibition of the parasympathetic nerve supply. If pethidine is to be given with atropine then only half the usual dose of atropine is required because pethidine itself has a slight atropine-like action. Pethidine is contraindicated in patients with severe liver disease and also in those patients receiving monoamine oxidase inhibitors. It should be remembered that morphine and its derivatives produce respiratory depression, but this is unlikely to cause problems as the dosage will be very low for an outpatient.

PHENOTHIAZINE DERIVATIVES

Antihistamines

These are sometimes used for premedication as, besides have an antiemetic action, they possess a hypnotic effect and potentiate the action of anaesthetics. An example of a suitable antihistamine is the phenothiazine derivative, promethazine hydrochloride (Phenergan, May and Baker), where the dosage for an adult would be 25 mg and that for a child over 5 years would be 10 mg. It may be prescribed as an elixir for young patients. Its duration of action is approximately 8 hours.

Another useful drug in this group, for paediatric use, is trimeprazine (Vallergan, May and Baker). The syrup forte contains 30 mg/5 ml and can be given up to 3 mg per kg body weight. Duration of action is 8 hours.

BENZODIAZEPINE DERIVATIVES

1. Chlordiazepoxide (Librium, Roche)

This drug is a diazepine derivative which exercises a selective depression of the central nervous system, unlike the barbiturates which cause generalized depression. Chlordiazepoxide is a very useful tranquillizer, with slight muscle-relaxant properties. It has the disadvantage that it may increase the effects of alcohol and therefore patients, particularly drivers, should be warned of this.

The dosage for an adult is 15–30 mg taken orally 1 hour before dental treatment or 10 mg for a child or elderly patient. Its duration of action is sufficient for dental treatment lasting up to 1 hour, although the central nervous system depression may be present for as long as 4 hours after administration.

2. Diazepam (Valium, Roche; Diazemuls, KabiVitrum)

Diazepam is a benzodiazepine tranquillizer, chemically similar to chlordiazepoxide. It reduces anxiety so that a patient is more relaxed and cooperative. He becomes slightly drowsy and more tolerant of pain, although there is no analgesic action. Reactions are slowed, speech becomes slightly slurred, and he may become mildly ataxic. There appears to be general depression of the central nervous system with muscle relaxation and some subsequent amnesia, which is advantageous, but there is no cardiac depression and no alteration in the blood pressure. The incidence of nausea with this drug is very low, but even so the manufacturers of diazepam (Roche Products Ltd) recommend that it should be used only if food has been withheld as for general anaesthesia.

Diazepam has a prolonged effect, which is partly due to its breakdown into active products. This problem is apparent with repeated administration giving a cumulative effect, or if an overdose is given. The duration of action of a drug dose is approximately 8 hours.

3. Lorazepam (Ativan, Wyeth)

Another benzodiazepine derivative with the advantage over diazepam that it is not broken down into active products. Its elimination is also faster. It is a more powerful drug and also may be used intravenously. For intravenous sedation, increments of 0·5 mg can be given up to a total of 4 mg.

4. Midazolam (Hypnovel, Roche)

A benzodiazepine which is more rapidly eliminated than either diazepam or lorazepam. Up to 7·5 mg can be given, in 2·1 mg increments intravenously, to the average adult.

INTRAVENOUS SEDATION

The careful use of intravenous sedation together with local analgesia facilitates outpatient dental treatment on many patients who would be too nervous or uncooperative to be treated other than under general anaesthesia.

The technique is basically intravenous premedication followed by local analgesia in order to carry out routine treatment such as conservation and extractions. The rationale behind this method is that the effect of intravenous premedication is more reliable than the oral route. The dosage required is about a quarter of that needed when the oral route is used, as the drugs are passed directly into the bloodstream and reach the brain in known amounts, whereas the results of oral administration are extremely variable as they depend on absorption of the drug through the gastrointestinal tract and metabolism in the liver. Even after calculating the normal dosage, such factors as the time of the last meal, its constituents and quantity, and the degree of apprehension of the patient, all make a vast difference to the sedation achieved. Because of these variables one patient may be rendered nearly unconscious by the administration of a normal dose whereas another will be little affected by three times that dosage. Similarly, the time of onset of sedation is unreliable. In one person it may be half an hour whereas in another little effect will be noticed for 2–3 hours, which may be long after the operation has finished. At this time the patient may

be homeward bound, when the sedation may cause considerable inconvenience and be potentially dangerous.

Because of the problems associated with oral premedication, intravenous techniques were introduced, an early method being that developed by the late Professor Niels B. Jorgensen. This used pentobarbitone sodium (sodium pentobarbitol, USP; Nembutal), pethidine and hyoscine (scopolamine), but this mixture depressed the respiratory and circulatory centres so much that occasionally prolonged postoperative drowsiness was a serious drawback. At the present time, the commonest drug used for intravenous sedation on dental patients is diazepam.

CHOICE OF PATIENTS

Intravenous sedation is unsuitable for children under 12, and also for pregnant patients, especially during the first trimester. It is an established medical principle that drugs should be administered in early pregnancy only when there are absolute indications.

Intravenous sedation is a technique which is particularly useful for treatment under these four headings.

1. To sedate the genuinely apprehensive and nervous patient

In these people the use of the technique encourages them to attend for treatment which they would otherwise avoid. The fact that the dentistry is performed under sedation permits a considerable increase in both the quality and quantity of work carried out at a single visit. The use of intravenous sedation also eliminates the strain which is imposed on a dental surgeon when operating on nervous patients.

2. Medical considerations

In the case of the mentally retarded patient the technique is of great value. It may also help to control the motor disturbances associated with nervous disorders such as cerebral palsy, where the patient may be of high intelligence but unable to keep still during treatment.

3. To control gagging reflexes

A patient may find it impossible to tolerate any foreign body within the mouth, even the taking of a bite-wing radiograph being difficult. In a few cases it is almost impossible to carry out dental treatment, the administration intraorally of an inferior dental nerve block, for instance, being too hazardous a procedure to attempt for fear of needle fracture. In these cases, the use of intravenous sedation transforms the patient from being involuntarily uncooperative to one who is readily amenable to treatment.

4. To control salivary secretions

A suitable drug to reduce salivary secretions can be administered with the other premedicants. This may be of considerable assistance in obtaining a dry field in which to operate.

CASE HISTORY OF PATIENT

It is important to take a careful case history prior to administering any drug intravenously or indeed orally, and if there is any feature in the case history which appears to be in any way unfavourable then the patient's physician must always be consulted.

When there is severe impairment of liver function, as may occur in advanced cirrhosis, then it is wise to avoid the administration of intravenous drugs as their elimination may be impaired and thus very deep sedation and delayed recovery experienced.

If the patient is taking hypnotics or tranquillizers, then these will potentiate the action of the intravenous premedicants. Similarly, alcoholism, drug addiction, cachexia, severe anaemia and hypotension may all modify the action of the drugs used. Should the case history disclose any of these conditions then either the intravenous sedation technique should be avoided or advice sought from the patient's medical practitioner before proceeding. When the administration of local analgesics is contraindicated, then this method of sedation should not be used.

PRECAUTIONS

Although it is unlikely that oxygen will be required, it should always be available together with the emergency resuscitation equipment which is to hand when general anaesthetics are given.

TECHNIQUE WITH DIAZEPAM

The route commonly employed for premedication with diazepam is intravenous and the dosage usually given varies between 10 and 20 mg for a healthy adult. The new formulation in a lipid emulsion (Diazemuls) is not irritant. It is supplied in 2-ml ampoules containing 10 mg. Up to 0·8 mg per kg bodyweight would be insufficient to cause loss of consciousness and therefore the amounts quoted for premedication appear to be safe. The rate of injection should not exceed 2·5 mg per 30 seconds and this rate of injection is continued until adequate sedation is achieved. The drug acts quickly, the onset of premedication taking 30–90 seconds.

Diazepam reduces muscle tone and thus the correct degree of sedation can be judged by such indications as the appearance of Verrill's sign. With this, the small sensitive muscles supplying the upper eyelid are relaxed to the extent that the eyelid droops until it is bisecting the iris. The dosage almost invariably falls between 0·15 and 0·3 mg per kg bodyweight and no more than 20 mg should be given to a large healthy male.

Diazepam reduces anxiety so that most patients are more relaxed and cooperative. The patient becomes slightly drowsy and more tolerant of pain, although there is no analgesic action. He is not confused or disorientated but reactions are slowed, speech becomes slightly slurred and he may become mildly ataxic. There appears to be general depression of the central nervous system with muscle relaxation and some subsequent amnesia, which is advantageous, but there is no cardiac depression and no alteration in the blood pressure.

On occasions, with slight overdose of diazepam, a patient may become totally disorientated and uncooperative, in which case the technique must be abandoned. The temptation of giving further doses in excess of 20 mg must be avoided, because diazepam may cause respiratory depression and loss of protective airway reflexes. Should a loss of consciousness occur, the patient must be laid flat, turned on his side and attention given to the patency of the airway. Oxygen 100 per cent should be given in these circumstances.

TECHNIQUE WITH PENTAZOCINE AND DIAZEPAM

Pentazocine (Fortral, Winthrop) is an allyl derivative of phenazocine and acts as a partial narcotic antagonistic analgesic intermediate between codeine and morphine. It has a low risk of producing dependency and does not produce the mental detachment of morphine. Frequently unpleasant hallucinations are reported with moderate dosages of pentazocine. Therefore, its use as the sole sedative drug does not compare favourably with diazepam. Brown et al. (1975) reported on the use of 30 mg of pentazocine intravenously with small (5 mg) increments of diazepam, care being taken not to administer an overdosage of diazepam as the respiratory depressant effect of the two drugs summates. The advantages of using pentazocine are that a smaller dose of diazepam is needed, recovery is slightly quicker, and possibly the pentazocine potentiates the analgesic action of the local analgesics. These advantages are probably too slight to warrant recommending this technique as being better than the simpler method of using diazepam as the sole intravenous agent.

POSTOPERATIVE CARE

Recovery from diazepam is usually fairly rapid with the dosages described above. The main effects will have worn off within ½ hour and the patient is usually fit to leave the surgery within 1½ hours to return home with an escort. The patient should be discharged only if accompanied by a responsible adult and, indeed, the operation should not have started without it being certain that an escort would be available. On no account should the patient be allowed to return to work or to drive or use machinery on the same day, also alcohol should be avoided as its action is potentiated. An occasional complication which has been reported is a secondary depression occurring 3–4 hours after administration of large >20 mg) doses of diazepam.

ADVANTAGES

1. It allays fear and anxiety, thus making the patient more relaxed and cooperative.
2. It raises the pain threshold.
3. The gag reflex is controlled, enabling one to operate in poorly accessible areas without disturbing the patient.
4. There is a considerable degree of postoperative amnesia, the patient remembering little of the proceedings on the following day.
5. The patient loses all sense of time and if asked after 2 hours for how long he feels he has been treated, will probably say 15–30 minutes. Long, difficult procedures can thus be undertaken without disturbing the patient.

DISADVANTAGES

1. The most important one is that the premedication generally lasts somewhat longer than the treatment.
2. Recovery facilities are essential.
3. The patient must be escorted by a responsible person.
4. The patient is unable to work or drive after treatment on the same day.

RELATIVE ANALGESIA

This is the term used to describe a means of sedation in which the conscious patient inhales a mixture of nitrous oxide, oxygen and air via a lightweight nosepiece.

Relative analgesia is considered to be part of stage one of the four stages of anaesthesia—stage two is the excitement stage, stage three is surgical anaesthesia and stage four is respiratory paralysis.

This technique was introduced about 1940, one of its early protagonists being Harry Langa. He found that patients receiving a low concentration of nitrous oxide and high concentrations of oxygen became more susceptible to suggestion, were relaxed and were completely cooperative. The semi-hypnotic aspect of suggestion was a very important part of the relative analgesia technique besides the inhalation of nitrous oxide. Although analgesia was not marked, the pain threshold was raised enough to tolerate minor discomfort without complaint, local analgesia injections being used as an adjunct when required. Other advantages are that nitrous oxide is very rapidly taken in and eliminated from the body, and that commonly the patients have some amnesia which makes them unaware postoperatively of any unpleasant aspects of their dental treatment.

Contraindications to relative analgesia include obstruction of the nasal airway, respiratory disease, disseminated sclerosis and psychiatric disease. The technique should not be used during the first trimester of pregnancy but thereafter is safe, provided care is taken to avoid any hypoxia.

There are machines designed specifically for the administration of relative analgesia, an example being the Quantiflex RA Mk II manufactured by Cyprane (*Fig.* 13.2). This has a minimum oxygen flow preset at 3 litres/min which achieves a minimum oxygen concentration of 23 volumes per cent in the mixed anaesthetic gases. There is also an automatic

cut-off of nitrous oxide flow should there be any failure in the oxygen supply. The air intake valve introduces room air automatically if the gas flow has stopped or the reservoir bag is depleted, and the possibility of a build-up of carbon dioxide occurring is eliminated by the use of a non-return valve behind the fresh gas outlet.

After treatment has been completed the patient is given pure oxygen to breathe for 2–3 minutes and then rests for 20–30 minutes, after which time he should be completely fit to leave the surgery and continue with normal activities.

HYPNOSIS

This method is sometimes of use in susceptible patients and the technique has been mentioned in Chapter 2.

The hypnotist's skill in quietly talking to a patient may be a useful way of calming a person even although not fully hypnotized. It is possible that a course in hypnosis would provide a dental surgeon with more insight into ways of reassuring and calming nervous patients.

CONCLUSION

Oral premedication is seldom worth using on healthy well-adjusted outpatients who are to have treatment done under local analgesia. However, when a patient is on continuous sedation therapy for a nervous disorder, a benefit may be derived from the physician prescribing an increased dose prior to dental treatment. Purely hypnotic drugs are not satisfactory premedicants as they have little effect in reducing apprehension. Instead they may produce a reduction in self-control which might be proportional to the hypnotic effect and, particularly with children, this would prevent any benefit being derived from their use.

If a patient's cooperation cannot be encouraged by discussion, then the operator may have to decide whether general anaesthesia should be used or whether the patient should be admitted to a hospital or nursing home where

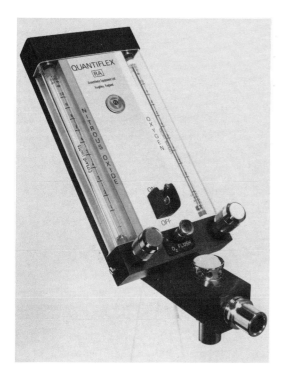

Fig. 13.2. The flowmeters of the Quantiflex machine for relative analgesia.

there will be no problems preoperatively if the dose of premedicant has induced drowsiness or sleep. Useful alternatives may be the employment of intravenous sedation techniques, relative analgesia or hypnosis. Of these alternative techniques, intravenous sedation is probably the most efficient.

REFERENCES AND FURTHER READING

Allen W. (1976) Relative analgesia. *Dent. Practice* **14**, 7.
Brown P. R. H., Main D. M. G. and Wood N. (1975) Intravenous sedation in dentistry. A study of 55 cases using pentazocine and diazepam. *Br. Dent. J.* **139**, 59.
Langa H. (1976) *Relative Analgesia in Dental Practice*, 2nd ed. Philadelphia, Saunders.

Chapter 14

COMPLICATIONS OCCURRING IN LOCAL ANALGESIA

Complications can arise from the injection of a local analgesic which may be due to the drugs used or the actual technique of injection. Whereas some complications may cause the patient little inconvenience, others may lead the operator into the Coroner's Court.

COMPLICATIONS ARISING FROM THE DRUGS OR CHEMICALS USED

Allergy and hypersensitivity

A patient may exhibit an allergic or hypersensitivity reaction to the local analgesic solution and this can be caused by any of the constituents such as the analgesic drug, vasoconstrictor, or even other ingredients such as bacteriostatic agents which have been added. Recent work has shown that the majority of reported allergies to lignocaine local anaesthetic solutions have been due to the paraben bacteriostatic agent and not to the actual lignocaine (Luebke and Walker, 1978; Lederman et al., 1980). These reactions are not fully understood but are thought to be due to a type of antigen–antibody reaction. The antigen is a chemical or drug, usually a protein or polysaccharide, which reacts with a substance known as an 'antibody', produced within the patient almost invariably as a result of a previous exposure to the antigen.

Hypersensitivity reactions cause tissue damage and may be grouped under four headings. Reactions of types I, II and III are termed 'immediate responses' which produce their maximum effect within about 4–8 hours and are due to serum antibodies. The type IV reaction is a 'delayed response', occurring after 24–48 hours due to interaction of antigen with sensitized T-lymphocytes.

Type I: anaphylactic hypersensitivity where the antigen reacts with the antibody IgE which is bound to mast cells and basophils causing the release of histamine and other chemical mediators which produce an inflammatory reaction.

Type II: antibody-dependent cytotoxic hypersensitivity where tissue damage occurs because the cells have antigen present on their surfaces which combines with antibody producing lysis and cell death.

Type III: immune complex-mediated hypersensitivity in which an antigen–antibody reaction involving blood vessels causes complement activation which in turn produces a leucotactic response. The leucocytosis causes ingestion of immune complexes and subsequent tissue damage due to the release of lysosomal enzymes.

Type IV: delayed-type hypersensitivity in which sensitized T-lymphocytes proliferate and cause tissue damage by releasing lymphokines.

In the case of local anaesthetics, the mechanism usually involves the small anaesthetic molecule acting as a hapten, that is to say it is not capable of exciting an immune reaction on its own, but does so by binding with and altering the stereochemical configuration of tissue proteins, such that the immune system comes to regard these proteins as 'foreign' antigens and acts in an appropriate way, usually by generating antibodies to these proteins and imitating a type I or III hypersensitivity reaction.

Of the drugs used to achieve local analgesia in dentistry the most common ones to produce reactions are procaine, cocaine and amethocaine. The incidence of allergic responses to procaine and related substances has been estimated as high as 6 per cent; however, lignocaine, as has been mentioned previously, and prilocaine are remarkably free from these side-effects.

An example of a type I reaction is the production of angioneurotic oedema (*Fig.* 14.1). This condition usually causes a rapidly developing swelling around the lips, tongue, eyes and occasionally other sites. The release of histamine produces a vasodilatation with oedema arising from the transudation of tissue fluid which is often transient and seldom persists for longer than 24 hours. The greatest danger may arise from oedema of the glottis which can cause respiratory obstruction.

The treatment of angioneurotic oedema is directed towards preventing further attacks by identifying the antigen responsible for initiating the reaction. The actual attack is usually relieved by antihistamine drugs such as preferably chlorpheniramine maleate (Piriton, Allen and Hanburys), the adult dosage being 10 mg given slowly intravenously, or promethazine hydrochloride (Phenergan, May and Baker) 25 mg intramuscularly, this latter preparation being

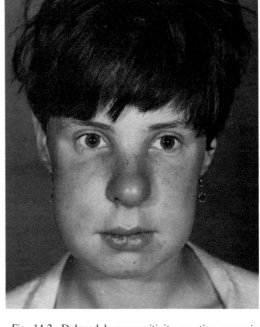

Fig. 14.2. Delayed hypersensitivity reaction occurring 24 hours after injection of procaine, producing an irritant skin rash and inflammation of the soft tissues.

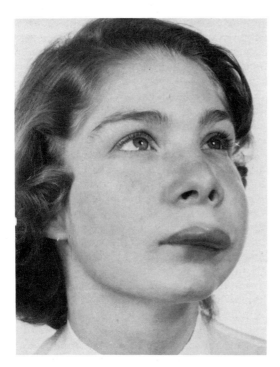

Fig. 14.1. Facial swelling typical of angioneurotic oedema. (Reproduced by courtesy of Dr J. F. Lockwood.)

not quite so efficient as it has less anti-inflammatory and greater sedative action. However, if the symptoms are very severe then intravenous hydrocortisone sodium succinate 100 mg or 0·5 ml of 1 : 1000 adrenaline should be given subcutaneously and oxygen administered. If these measures fail and respiratory obstruction is likely to endanger life, then a crico-thyrotomy needle such as the Abelsohn pattern should be inserted or a tracheostomy performed.

Delayed hypersensitivity reactions due to allergy to a drug are not uncommon and indeed some drugs invoke this reaction fairly frequently. This usually takes several hours or days to appear and commonly produces an irritant urticarial rash which may cover a large area of the skin (*Fig.* 14.2). There may be pyrexia, with lymphadenopathy and arthralgia, and rarely there may be oral ulceration. The treatment of this condition should be with anti-histamines, and in very severe cases cortico-steroids may be given with antibiotics to treat any secondary infection which might arise if ulceration has occurred.

Allergic dermatitis

It should be remembered that in addition to the patient, the operator may also become allergic to the drugs he uses, and indeed there are many cases of dental surgeons who are unable to use drugs such as amethocaine because of this.

When inflammation of the skin occurs due to allergy then the condition is termed an *allergic dermatitis*. If the allergen is carried to the skin via the blood or lymph the condition is *intrinsic* and if contacted externally it is *extrinsic*. This latter type is also known as a *contact dermatitis* or *dermatitis venenata*. In this condition a lesion is produced at a localized site such as a finger-tip after repeated contact with the causative drug (*Fig.* 14.3). Contact dermatitis is a type IV

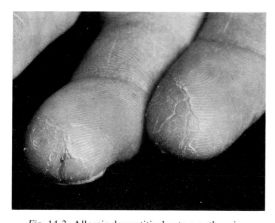

Fig. 14.3. Allergic dermatitis due to amethocaine.

hypersensitivity reaction which is cell-mediated and delayed in onset. The drugs usually act as haptens binding with tissue protein which is then recognized as 'foreign' by the dermal macrophages, Langerhans' cells, which are responsible for presenting the allergen to the T-cells. These T-lymphocytes release a variety of lymphokines which are responsible for the local inflammatory response which produces the local tissue destruction. At this site there may be an initial irritation of the skin followed by reddening, vesicle or bullae formation, and then ulceration of those which get infected. The lesions may become very chronic if there is repeated contact with the causative drug. If the operator must persist with the use of the particular drug then the hands should be protected by wearing rubber gloves.

Idiosyncrasy

Idiosyncrasy is a rare complication which may occur as a reaction to any drug and arises because a patient has an individual susceptibility. This susceptibility means that quite a small dose of the drug may produce symptoms associated with an overdosage. In local analgesia, idiosyncrasy may be due either to the vasoconstrictor or the analgesic drug. This situation is sometimes rather difficult to assess because it may be confused with syncope. However, if there is any doubt then the safest procedure is to discontinue the injection and postpone dental treatment. Should the patient remain collapsed then oxygen must be administered. In severe cases where cerebral irritation occurs leading to convulsions then the patient should be protected to avoid the risk of injury, for example inserting a pad of gauze between the teeth to prevent tongue-biting and by cushioning the head to avoid it striking the floor. At the same time the slow intravenous administration of diazepam up to a maximum of 20 mg may overcome the muscle spasms, the dosage for elderly patients being up to a maximum of 10 mg. Diazepam is marketed in ampoules containing 5 mg per ml. With reactions of this severity, the patient should be admitted to hospital as an emergency for sedation under medical supervision. At a later date, it would be wise to warn the patient who has had a severe idiosyncratic reaction that the causative drug must be avoided. At the same time is would be desirable to write to the patient's medical practitioner and give him details of the episode to warn him of the risk, With the patient who has merely felt faint then, if there is anything in the previous history to suggest that this reaction could have been due to an idiosyncrasy, small test doses of various local analgesics should be administered subcutaneously to assess whether the reaction was due to a particular drug. Usually it is found that this type of reaction was in fact a faint or syncope, although death has occurred due to idiosyncrasy to a normal dose of 2 per cent lignocaine.

Reactions to the vasoconstrictor are often considered to be due to either idiosyncrasy or toxicity from an overdosage. Certain of the vasoconstrictors such as adrenaline and noradrenaline are naturally occurring hormones and therefore would be unlikely to produce true idiosyncrasy. Some of the adverse responses noted after their administration have probably been due to simple fainting, although there have been a few reports of what may have been true idiosyncrasy to adrenaline.

Another explanation of adverse reactions to adrenaline and noradrenaline is that there is a particular group of healthy adults possessing a nervous, artistic temperament who react to stress situations—such as visits to the dental surgery—by having an excessive outpouring of adrenaline into the blood. Hence when a normal dosage of local analgesic containing adrenaline is injected, the cumulative effect on the patient resembles that of an overdose. An excess of vasopressor may result in tachycardia, palpitations, tremors, dyspnoea and hypertension, or may imitate a mild overdosage of analgesic by producing cerebral stimulation.

Skin testing

Skin testing for idiosyncrasy or allergy may be performed as follows. The skin of the flexor aspect of the forearm is usually the most convenient site and if the patient is right-handed then the left arm is used. This skin should not be sterilized, as antiseptics temporarily impair its ability to react to test doses. The site should be cleaned with mild soap and water and then marked with ink so that the test areas may be identified. Approximately 0·01–0·02 ml of solution is injected intradermally, that is into the skin and not beneath it, so that a small bleb is formed. Besides injecting the various local analgesic solutions, a control injection of pyrogen-free water or saline should be made for comparative purposes. During these injections it may be possible to note whether the patient has any idiosyncratic reaction to a particular drug. After a period of 48 hours the patient's forearm should be inspected to note whether there is any erythema or weal formation.

Nasal testing

Another method of testing for idiosyncrasy or allergy is by challenging the nasal mucosa with the drug in question by applying it to the surface of the nasal epithelium. The patient is tilted back at approximately 45°, the drug instilled, and the nose examined using a nasal speculum at 2-minute intervals. If the drug is provoking an allergic reaction then in severe cases the nasal mucosa becomes grossly erythematous and swollen to produce complete unilateral nasal obstruction. This reaction reaches its maximum within 30 minutes and there should be no general symptoms. The nasal blockage is quickly reversed by the application of 0·5 per cent ephedrine sulphate nasal drops.

It has been reported that both intradermal and nasal testing occasionally gives false-negatives, as the local anaesthetics can act as haptens or a metabolite may be the antigen in delayed reactions, so that extensive and painful lesions can result from tests.

Contaminated solutions

Complications may arise from the injection of solutions which have become contaminated.

Some dental surgeons, possibly through thoughtlessness, use part of a cartridge on one patient and then later use the remainder on another. This practice must be condemned because of the risk of producing cross-infection. When an injection is given there is a back-pressure exerted by the tissues so that fluid flows back into the analgesic solution. If some of this solution is later injected into another patient then there is the risk of inoculating him with any infection which the original patient may have been carrying. The only safe rule is for all partly used analgesic cartridges to be discarded immediately a patient has left the surgery.

Another potentially dangerous method of contamination of a cartridge was described in Chapter 6, where a case report was quoted of complications following the entry of antiseptic into an analgesic solution. It is easy to appreciate how a similar type of mishap might arise in dental work.

A further risk occurs because a dental surgeon or nurse may use empty cartridges to store solutions other than analgesics, sometimes without even bothering to relabel them. This dangerous habit frequently leads to the incorrect solution being injected into a patient, sometimes with disastrous results. Substances which have been injected by mistake include phenol, mercury, ammonia, trichloracetic acid, halothane, whisky and lighter fuel. In recent years hydrogen peroxide, which is commonly used for irrigating root canals, has become the most frequent offender.

Overdosage

Very occasionally overdosage may occur due to the injection of too large an amount of local analgesic. This is most likely when an inexperienced operator makes repeated inaccurate injections and, in his enthusiasm to obtain satisfactory analgesia, forgets just how much solution has been used.

Another cause of overdosage is the inadvertent intravascular injection, hence the need for routine aspiration prior to injecting. Relative overdosage is more likely to occur when normal metabolism of the drug is impaired, such as occurs in patients with cardiovascular failure, and hepatic or renal disease.

With most of the local analgesic drugs administered by injection, mild overdosage results in cerebral stimulation which may mask evidence of medullary depression. If a large overdosage occurs then the cortical effects are absent and the vital centres are affected, causing respiratory depression or cardiac arrest. The symptoms of overdosage may progress from light-headedness, dizziness, headache, nausea and vomiting to the development of a confused state in which the patient may be euphoric or apprehensive, with twitching of the face and difficulty with speech and dysphagia. From this stage the patient becomes disorientated and comatose with muscular twitching spreading to the limbs and eventually leading to convulsions. This is a dangerous period because the convulsions may interfere with respiration and lead to hypoxia. At the onset of this stage the blood pressure and pulse rate may both be raised, but with the development of respiratory depression and hypoxia, myocardial impairment ensues, leading to a fall in blood pressure and cardiac arrest. The treatment of overdosage is directed to maintaining an adequate oxygen supply to the brain.

Treatment of overdosage

1. Put the patient on his back with the head as low as possible.

2. Inflate the lungs with oxygen, with or without laryngeal intubation, depending upon whether someone skilled at intubating is available. The administration of external artificial respiration is unsuccessful on a chest which is convulsing.

3. Give a 'sleep dose' (possibly up to about 20 mg in increments of 2·5 mg of 0·5 per cent, 5 mg/ml solution) of diazepam (Valium, Roche) slowly intravenously to stop convulsions.

4. If respiration ceases do *not* give nikethamide (Coramine, Ciba) as this will restart convulsions. The use of respiratory stimulants will be ineffective because the local analgesics have a stimulant action and the depression of the respiratory centre which has occurred is the result of their previous overstimulation.

5. Continue inflation of the lungs with oxygen until spontaneous respirations occur.

6. Restore cardiac output with carefully controlled intravenous fluids and the cautious use of positive ionotropic agents may be of value. Occasional reports of cardiac arrhythmias, and particularly heart block, have led to attempts at temporary cardiac pacing to restore sufficient cardiac output until the excess local anaesthetic has been cleared.

Fortunately, these complications usually only arise as a result of mistakes, such as the intravenous overdose of lignocaine in cardiac use, the commonest error being the use of 2-g intravenous boluses instead of an intended 200-mg bolus. The standard loading dose of lignocaine is 50–100 mg intravenously when used for controlling ventricular arrhythmias, followed by a continuous infusion. Bearing this in mind, it should be very unusual to achieve huge overdoses by dental injections using solutions such as 2 per cent lignocaine with an added vasoconstrictor which delays its absorption.

When administering any drug, the maximum safe dosage must always be related to the bodyweight of the patient and to his general health and age. The dosages quoted assume that the patient is a fit adult with a bodyweight of 70 kg (11 stone). The size of the doses must be reduced for the elderly, debilitated and very young patients. Further information regarding dosages for children is given in Chapter 13.

COMPLICATIONS ASSOCIATED WITH INJECTION TECHNIQUES

These will be considered in their likely chronological order.

Fainting

The most common complication of an injection is that the patient may feel faint. He becomes pale, sweating, cold, feels unwell and may lose consciousness. This is a very common complication and should not be confused with the possibility of a hypersensitivity to synthetic adrenaline which, if it exists, is extremely rare.

Fainting or syncope frequently occurs because the patient is frightened at the thought of receiving an injection. This nervousness may be aggravated because he has been suffering from toothache causing disturbed sleep. This is particularly so if the patient is unaccustomed to dental treatment, has not got a regular practitioner and consequently has not the usual confidence in the operator. All these factors combine to increase the patient's apprehension.

It is sometimes stated that a patient receiving an injection should have eaten recently in order that the blood-sugar level will be satisfactory, and if he has not eaten then it is a wise precaution to administer a sweetened drink such as fruit squash containing glucose. In normal people, the homeostatic mechanism controlling blood-glucose concentrations does not allow the glucose to fall to hypoglycaemic levels for at least 48 hours. There is no strong evidence that vasovagal attacks are associated with hypoglycaemia and therefore the practice of recommending glucose drinks to such patients is probably of doubtful value, apart from the not unimportant psychological benefit. Although vasoconstrictors such as adrenaline and nor-adrenaline do raise the blood-sugar level, the small amounts which may be present in a local analgesic solution are unlikely to have much effect.

Treatment of syncope

If a patient does feel faint then the head should be lowered, either by placing it between the knees, which may be difficult or even impossible if the patient is obese, or preferably tilting the dental chair back so that the head is lower than the feet. As fainting is due to an inadequate blood supply to the brain, this helps to restore the cerebral circulation. The dental surgeon or the dental nurse should remain close to the patient so that there is no chance of the patient falling out of the chair in the event of consciousness being lost. This is extremely important as cerebral anoxia may lead to convulsions.

All dental chairs should be made so that the patient can quickly be placed flat for the institution of resuscitation, preferably with the head lower than the heart and the feet raised. If this is not possible then the cumbersome procedure of lifting the patient up and putting him on the floor becomes necessary. This is a dangerous manoeuvre because if the patient is unconscious and has had extractions performed, then it is almost certain that his head has to be raised and blood or fluid may enter the trachea. One-piece chairs are unsatisfactory as the back rest cannot be lowered separately, and with chairs that are electrically controlled, unless the back rest can be let down by a simple movement, the electric method of lowering the back is likely to waste valuable time.

It is very easy for the early signs of respiratory and cardiac failure to be confused with those of a simple faint. If the patient does not immediately respond to resuscitative measures then avoid wasting precious time and assume that acute collapse has occurred. The management of this is described in the section on 'Cardiac Arrest' (see below).

If the unconscious patient has any tight clothing such as a collar or belt which may impede respiration, then this should be loosened. Check the pulse and respirations, and if recovery is not immediate then the airway should be cleared by removing any foreign body such as a loose denture, and pushing the mandible into a protruded position to bring the tongue forwards in order to maintain a patent airway. Oxygen, which must always be available, should then be administered. If the recovery to consciousness has taken more than 5 minutes or the patient feels unwell, then he should be seen by a doctor in case there is an underlying medical condition.

Usually the patient rapidly recovers from a faint and frequently, on being reassured by the kindness and efficiency of the operator and nurse, is willing to continue treatment. If the injection was for the purpose of achieving analgesia to relieve pain then it is probably best to proceed, as the sooner the treatment is completed then the sooner the patient's apprehension is allayed, and thus the likelihood of a further faint is lessened. If it is impossible to continue, then the patient should be given another appointment; however, there is the risk of syncope recurring at a subsequent visit unless preventative measures are taken. These include such items as advising the patient to have a meal beforehand, and at the next visit taking especial care to keep the patient calm. If the patient's head is kept low by having the dental chair tilted back then fainting is much less likely. Probably the most important factor in preventing fainting is a reassuring chair-side manner.

Other types of collapse

Some other types of collapse may occur in the dental surgery and therefore need to be considered, although they may be unassociated with injection techniques.

These emergencies include cardiac arrest, attacks of angina pectoris, coronary thrombosis, respiratory obstruction and arrest, cerebrovascular accident, epileptic fits, diabetic and hypoglycaemic comas, and steroid and thyroid crises. Their treatment usually requires hospitalization and therefore an ambulance should be summoned.

1. Cardiac arrest

Cardiac arrest is a very rare emergency but prompt action can save life and therefore it is essential to know the treatment of this complication. Cardiac arrest is equivalent to 'unexpected death' or 'acute collapse', and when it occurs the patient may suddenly start fitting and then lapse into deep unconsciousness when the diagnosis should be sought by feeling for arterial pulses. At first respiration may be slow and stertorous with absence of respiratory effort and then dilated pupils are late signs of cardiac arrest. Absence of the carotid or radial pulses are confirmatory signs. However, if the dental surgeon is not sure whether cardiac arrest has occurred, then he should assume that

it has and take the necessary action because no permanent harm will arise from this. 'Better a living mistake than a dead certainty.' The dental surgeon has 3 minutes in which to act before the patient suffers permanent brain damage, so if there is another person present such as the dental nurse, then this person should note the time and call it out at half-minute intervals. The treatment is simple (*Fig.* 14.4): first the patient is quickly laid flat on a firm surface, the exact time of the arrest noted, and then one sharp blow to the praecordium (that part of the chest wall overlying the heart) is given as sometimes this will restart the heart. But do not waste time.

If cardiac arrest is likely to be due to acute hypoxia then:

A. Airway: This is maintained by holding the chin forwards and if possible inserting an airway such as the Brook or a Resusitube (*Fig.* 14.5).

B. Breathing: This may be performed either by the dental surgeon placing his mouth over the patient's open mouth and carrying out rapid, deep, forced expirations and at the same time squeezing the patient's nose to occlude the nostrils or, if an anaesthetic machine is available with a bag, the oxygen can be forcibly insufflated into the lungs under direct pressure by squeezing the bag. If an anaesthetist is present, or if the dental surgeon has the necessary skill, an endotracheal tube should be inserted but time must not be wasted. Facilities for administering oxygen to a patient are essential for all dental surgeries.

C. Closed cardiac massage: The dental surgeon then administers a very sharp blow to the praecordium. This mechanical stimulus often starts the heart beating. If this is unsuccessful place the flat palmar aspect of both hands over the lower end of the sternum and compress the chest about 4 cm (1½ in), 70 times a minute.

This massage should produce a palpable carotid pulse which must be maintained to avoid permanent brain damage. If the patient's legs are raised then this will increase the venous return.

If cardiac arrest is unlikely to be due to acute hypoxia, then start with external cardiac massage before beginning artificial respiration as the brain is more susceptible to ischaemia than to hypoxia.

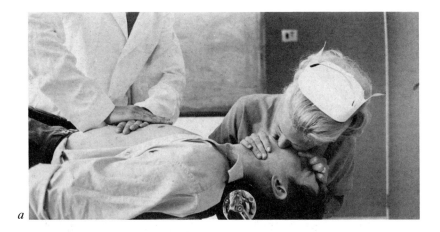

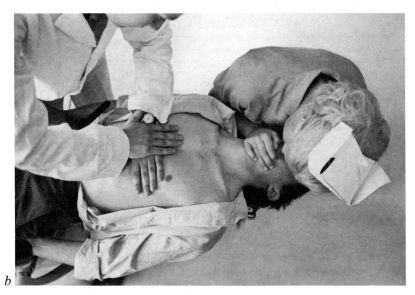

Fig. 14.4. Treatment of cardiac and respiratory arrest. The patient has been tilted so that his head is below the heart. Note that the nurse holds the mandible forward to clear the airway, at the same time as she watches the chest moving during mouth-to-mouth respiration. The lower picture (*b*) shows pressure being applied to the lower end of the sternum during cardiac massage.

If the dental surgeon is single-handed when this emergency arises, then he should alternate five impulses to the heart with one forced expiration into the patient's lungs. If another person is available then one person should maintain the respiration and the other the cardiac massage, both of which should be continued for as long as possible, and medical assistance summoned urgently. If the treatment is unsuccessful the dental surgeon should realize that nothing more could have been done for the patient, but if treatment had not been attempted then the coroner may have grounds for levelling criticism at him.

If a defibrillator is available even in the absence of a monitor, electroconversion should be considered as soon as possible, since the success rate is time-dependent and even if the

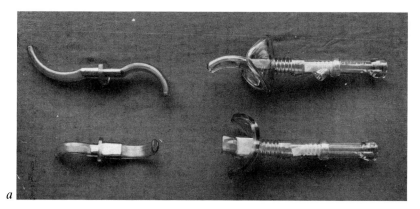

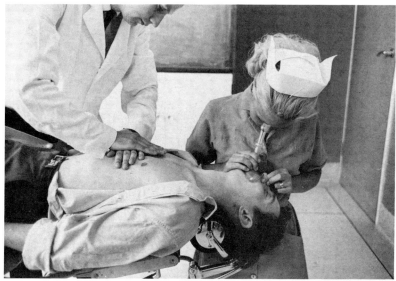

Fig. 14.5. *a,* Varieties of airway. The combined Guedel airway on the left and the Brook pattern with non-return valve on the right. The lower pair are for use with children. *b,* Artificial respiration using the Brook airway. Note the fingers occluding the nostrils.

heart is asystolic, no harm will arise from early electroconversion. Many ambulances now carry defibrillators, and ECG monitors.

It is also important to establish an intravenous access route at the earliest opportunity. However, this should only be done where there are sufficient practitioners available to ensure that the basic support manoeuvres are continued.

2. Angina pectoris

This causes a constricting pain around the chest which may radiate into the neck, down the left arm, occasionally down the right and sometimes into the jaws. This is usually brought on by exertion but may occur at rest when anxiety and excitement are predisposing factors. The attack is relieved by placing a 0·5-mg tablet of glyceryl trinitrate under the tongue and allowing it to disintegrate without swallowing. Alternatively, an aerosol spray of glyceryl trinitrate may be used which gives a metered dose of about 0·4 mg which should be sprayed on the oral mucosa, preferably on or under the tongue. Nitrous oxide and oxygen mixtures such as Entonox may also be useful and are likely to be available to some dental practitioners. The patient is often more comfortable standing up than lying down.

3. Coronary thrombosis

This causes a severe chest pain due to myocardial ischaemia and dyspnoea, the attack frequently occurring at rest and being of sudden onset. Characteristically the patient is mentally well orientated with a sense of impending death, which unfortunately often occurs very quickly. He will have an anxious, ashen appearance and be severely shocked, with lowered blood pressure and sometimes an irregular pulse. The immediate treatment is to maintain the airway, give oxygen if the patient is unconscious, make him rest if he is conscious, and, if available, give intravenous diamorphine (heroin) 2·5–5 mg. This may be administered in combination with an antiemetic such as prochlorperazine 12·5 mg intravenously. If there is evidence of left ventricular failure leading to pulmonary oedema, then an intravenous bolus of frusemide, 40–80 mg, should be administered.

4. Respiratory obstruction

In this emergency the patient coughs or chokes, becomes cyanosed, uses the accessory muscles of respiration and may collapse. The treatment is urgent and consists of clearing foreign bodies such as dentures, blood or mucus from the mouth and pharynx, sucking out the throat, clearing the airway, pushing the mandible forward to bring the tongue forward with it, and administering oxygen. If this has not relieved the condition and it is thought that obstruction may be due to an inhaled foreign body, then the Heidbrink manoeuvre should be employed. This involves standing behind the patient, placing ones arms around the chest and sharply compressing the chest in order to cause a sudden rise in intrathoracic pressure which is often sufficient to dislodge a foreign body. If obstruction persists, then insert a cricothyrotomy needle through the cricothyroid membrane or perform an emergency tracheostomy. Unless the airway is restored within about 3 minutes, irreversible brain damage will occur. If a cricothyrotomy needle has been inserted then it should be removed after 12 hours and if necessary an elective tracheostomy done. Ideally it should not be necessary to leave a cricothyrotomy needle in situ for 12 hours as the patient should have been transferred to hospital for bronchoscopic removal of the foreign body.

5. Respiratory arrest

This intervenes if respiratory obstruction is not relieved or it can occur as a sequel to damage to the respiratory centre, this in turn frequently being due to cerebral hypoxia following cardiac arrest. The patient becomes flaccid, cyanosed and his pupils are widely dilated. The treatment has been described under the management of cardiac arrest and is directed towards maintaining the airway and supplying adequate oxygen. This latter treatment may be done with mouth-to-mouth respiration or the use of an airway or endotracheal tube with positive-pressure resuscitation using a bag such as the Ambu type.

6. Cerebrovascular accident

This condition includes hypertensive intracerebral haemorrhage, cerebral embolism, caroticovertebral insufficiency and subarachnoid haemorrhage. There may be initial symptoms such as giddiness, headache and paraesthesia in the limbs of one side, followed by the rapid onset of deep coma in the case of cerebral or subarachnoid haemorrhage, with unilateral paralysis. The face is flushed and sweating and the pupils usually dilate and may be unequal, with the larger one being on the affected side. The pulse slows, respiration is stertorous and muscles relax with incontinence of faeces and urine. With a cerebral thrombosis the onset often occurs without any profound disturbance of consciousness. However, if the patient becomes unconscious, then the maintenance of the airway is essential and this may necessitate removing vomitus with a sucker to prevent respiratory obstruction. The further treatment is to arrange for the patient's transference by ambulance to hospital.

7. Epilepsy

In grand mal the patient frequently has an aura or warning and hence may be able to protect himself before the fit. During the attack the patient may let out a cry before falling down.

The patient then has a tonic spasm lasting about 30 seconds followed by clonic convulsions during which the patient may involuntarily micturate and defaecate. These latter signs help to differentiate an epileptic attack from any form of hysterical display. During the convulsion the epileptic may injure himself and this an hysteric is most unlikely to do. Following the convulsions, the attack passes into a coma stage which gradually changes to natural sleep.

In petit mal the patient suddenly becomes unconscious with glazed eyes but no convulsions. This type of attack may last only a few seconds.

The treatment of an epileptic attack is directed towards preventing the patient injuring himself. Frequently there is a risk of the tongue being badly bitten and this can be stopped by placing a suitable pack between the patient's teeth. Prolonged epileptic seizures are treated with intravenous diazepam.

It should be remembered that all local anaesthetic drugs are cerebral stimulants and that uncontrolled epileptics have a reduced threshold to cerebral irritation, leading to convulsions.

8. Diabetes

This is a very common disease, it being estimated that there are about 250 000 diabetics in the UK. The most important complications that may occur are those of coma, associated either with raised blood-sugar level due to insulin lack, or with lowered blood sugar due to relative insulin overdosage.

Diabetic coma due to hyperglycaemia is usually of gradual onset. The early symptoms are lassitude, tiredness, breathlessness on exertion and nausea. It progresses so that the patient becomes drowsy and comatose with air hunger causing the respirations to increase in frequency and depth. The breath smells of acetone. There are signs of dehydration such as inelasticity of the skin, dryness of the tongue and weakness of the pulse. The patient requires large doses of insulin and should be hospitalized. Also of importance, the patient requires major volumes of fluid replacement and careful electrolyte balance.

Hypoglycaemic coma is more common than diabetic coma and is due to an overdose of insulin. It usually occurs about an hour or so after a dose of insulin if there has been no subsequent food or about 4 hours afterwards if the insulin has been followed by an inadequate meal. The patient becomes weak, pale, sweating, with a rapid pulse and shallow respiration, and can be treated by giving him oral sugar or glucose. If the condition is not recognized then the patient will become disorientated, have muscular tremors, and may have convulsions followed by collapse and coma. If the patient is unconscious and cannot swallow voluntarily then intravenous glucose is the treatment of choice. In emergency, 1 mg of glucagon dissolved in 1 ml of its special diluent may be injected either intramuscularly or subcutaneously and will arouse most patients sufficiently for them to take sugar by mouth. A less safe alternative, provided that the glycogen reserves are still present, is to inject 0·5 ml of 1:1000 adrenaline subcutaneously as this may restore consciousness so that sugar may be given orally.

9. Steroid crisis

This may lead to collapse in a patient who has been on steroid therapy, especially long-term treatment on high dosages where atrophy of the adrenal cortex has occurred. The signs and symptoms of the collapse resemble those of a faint and include a thready pulse with hypotension and frequently fever. There may be peripheral vascular collapse causing cyanosis of the extremities and the patient may vomit. He should be treated by laying him flat, keeping him at a comfortable temperature and establishing an intravenous access route. With this in place, then 100 mg hydrocortisone hemisuccinate is required initially to combat shock, following which it is essential to ensure fluid replacement.

10. Thyroid crisis

This may rarely be precipitated by the anxiety arising from dental treatment. The patient becomes very restless, disorientated and semiconscious with a rapid, thready pulse and fever. This collapse may lead to cardiac failure and the patient should be transferred to hospital for emergency treatment.

Mechanical problems

1. Breakage of the analgesic cartridge

This may occur if there is excessive resistance to the flow of solution into the tissues. The most common occasion is when an attempt is made to inject too rapidly during the administration of a palatal injection, the mucosa being extremely firmly bound down to the underlying bone. If the cartridge glass breaks then care should be taken that all broken pieces are removed from the mouth so that there is no risk of them being ingested or cutting the patient.

2. Breakage of the syringe needle

Another complication which may occur is the breakage of a needle. Fortunately the modern

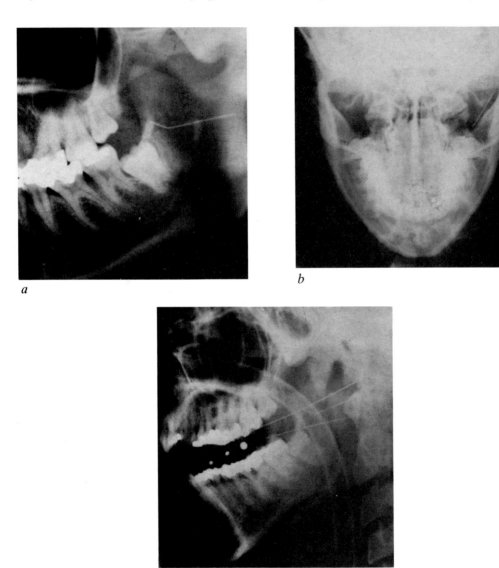

a *b* *c*

Fig. 14.6. Most needle fractures occur during an inferior dental injection. When this happens radiographs are taken in two different planes to locate the broken pieces (*a, b*). Radiopaque localizers may be inserted to further localize the retained fragment (*c*).

type is strong and flexible so that fracture is very rare although it is a particular hazard of the intraosseous injection.

Frazer-Moodie (1958) reported that the commonest cause of breakage was the use of an old needle, or a needle which had been bent and then straightened out again. His opinion was that if a needle was bent accidentally it should be discarded. The authors believe that all types of syringe needles should be discarded after they have been used for one patient because it is impossible to ensure that their lumina are satisfactorily cleaned and sterilized. With the advent of disposable needles there is no valid reason why this ideal should not be realized.

To avoid the accidental breakage of a needle it should never be buried into the tissues up to the hub and at least 6 mm (¼ in) of it should remain visible. For this reason a short needle must never be used for administering an inferior dental nerve block. Another common cause of breakage is the needle being jerked by a sudden or unexpected movement of the patient. When giving injections it is wise to have a small pair of curved Spencer-Wells or Mosquito artery forceps at hand so that if the needle breaks and the broken end is visible in the tissues, then without shifting the gaze, or the steadying finger, the operator can pick up the forceps and grasp the broken end of the needle to remove it. When the patient moves or swallows, then the broken fragment may shift deeper into the tissues and out of sight. If the broken needle end remains in the tissues then the patient should be transferred to the care of an oral surgeon for its removal. It is advisable to send the piece of needle remaining in the syringe and also an intact needle of a similar type so that he may assess the size of the broken fragment.

The oral surgeon will obtain radiographs in several planes to show the position of the broken needle (*Fig.* 14.6). Before arranging to remove it in theatre under an endotracheal general anaesthetic, he may use a radio-opaque localizer or other needles to help pinpoint the site of the retained fragment. Fraser-Moodie recommends the use of an electric or electronic locator in addition to localizers or pilot needles. An instrument such as the Berman locator will emit a sound which alters as its probe approaches the broken needle and this greatly facilitates the search.

The reasons for not leaving the broken fragment embedded in the tissues (*Fig.* 14.7) are:

1. The fragment is mobile and may travel quite a long way in the tissues, possibly to a position where it might be dangerous.

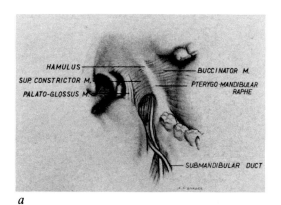

a

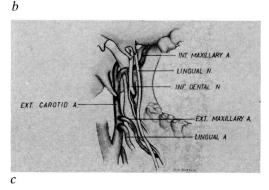

b

c

Fig. 14.7. Structures which may be encountered when removing a needle broken during the administration of an inferior dental nerve block. *a*, Superficial structures. *b*, Deeper structures. It is at this point that most broken needles are recovered. *c*, Vessels and nerves of the region. (Reproduced from W. Fraser-Moodie (1958) *Br. Dent. J.* **105**, 79.)

2. Psychological effect—worrying about 'something stuck in the throat'.

3. The fragment may induce scarring which could lead to trismus, dysphagia or pain.

4. The fragment may rupture a vessel.

Damage to the tissues

Tissue damage caused by the syringe needle may produce a wide variety of complications.

1. Vascular complications

a. Arterial irritation: If, during the injection, the needle touches an artery without penetrating the vessel wall, there may be a momentary discomfort often accompanied by blanching of the skin or mucous membrane. This vasoconstriction is due to spasm occurring in the muscular layer of the vessel, the tunica media, either because of direct stimulation of the muscle fibres or due to irritation of the sympathetic nerve plexus surrounding the vessel.

b. Intravascular injection: Should the analgesic be injected into a vessel accidentally, then the patient may develop a tachycardia and feel faint, with the added complication that the injection may fail to produce analgesia and overdosage may occur. It has been reported that intravascular injections occur in at least 5 per cent of injections, being least for infiltration techniques, more frequent for inferior dental nerve blocks, and most frequent for posterior superior dental injections, where the pterygoid venous plexus is closely related to the needle. Bishop (1983) records an incidence of 15·4 per cent positive aspirations in a total of 642 inferior dental nerve blocks administered to children between the ages of 7 and 16 years, suggesting that they run a greater risk of receiving intravascular injections while at the same time being more likely to receive relative overdoses.

The use of an aspirating syringe is mandatory because accidental injection of local analgesic solution into a blood vessel can be avoided if an aspirating syringe is used and the plunger withdrawn to check whether blood enters the cartridge prior to injection. If blood is visible in the cartridge, then the needle should be withdrawn a little so that its point is no longer in the vessel. Untoward reactions occurred in only about 10

per cent of all cases where a vessel had been entered and the analgesic solution was injected at a rate of less than 1 ml per minute. The lack of adverse reactions may have been due to the slow rate of injection or because of some apparently positive aspirations occurring where a vessel had been damaged, for example by nicking the vessel wall, or because part of the needle bevel was actually outside the vessel (*Fig.* 14.8).

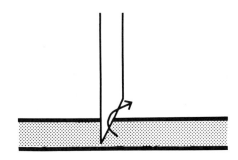

Fig. 14.8. Intravascular injection in which only part of the bevel of the needle is within the vessel. The arrow shows how bleeding may occur into the tissues.

It is obviously undesirable for local analgesic solutions to be accidentally injected intravascularly and therefore an aspirating syringe must always be used. It has been reported that toxicity following intravascular injections can be 200 times as high as when the analgesic is properly administered.

c. Haemorrhage occurring into the tissues: Commoner complications are associated with the trauma caused by the passage of the needle through the tissues during the injection. If the needle damages a vessel wall then bleeding into the tissues may occur (*Fig.* 14.8). This is most frequent when injecting in the region of the posterior superior dental nerve because, if the needle point is not kept close to the bone, there is the likelihood of trauma to the wall of one of the many vessels of the pterygoid venous plexus (*Fig.* 14.9). This damage shows itself by a rapidly developing swelling of the face due to the formation of a haematoma within the tissues. This may take a week or two to disperse and during that period there will be some trismus with discoloration or bruising of the skin. An explanation should be given to the patient to avoid any misapprehension regarding

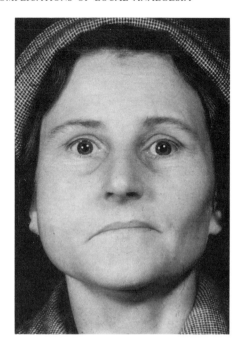

Fig. 14.9. This patient rapidly developed a haematoma on the right side of the face following a posterior superior dental injection.

his appearance. Other sites at which vessels are likely to be traumatized are in the pterygo-mandibular space and at the mental and infra-orbital foramina. Damage to blood vessels at this latter site may give the patient a 'black eye'.

No treatment is necessary, although some consider that the administration of a drug such as hyaluronidase, chymotrypsin or strepto-dornase might aid the more rapid dispersion of the bruising. If it is thought that the haematoma is likely to become infected then an antibiotic should be prescribed.

2. Nervous complications

a. Injury to a nerve: Occasionally during a nerve block injection, usually for the inferior dental and lingual nerves, the patient experiences a sudden pain which is commonly described as an 'electric shock' or resembling 'pins and needles' in the region supplied by the nerve and the onset of analgesia is particularly rapid. This combination of events means that the injection has been very accurate and the needle has touched the nerve, and in some cases damaged it. If the nerve has been damaged in

this way then occasionally anaesthesia persists for weeks or even months and on very rare occasions the damage may be permanent. Usually time heals and no treatment other than reassurance is required.

b. Facial nerve paralysis: Another complication which may arise during the administration of an inferior dental nerve block is facial paralysis which results in the patient being unable to smile or show the teeth when asked to do so. The cause of this complication is analgesic solution reaching the facial nerve, which may occur if the needle is inserted deeper than the posterior border of the vertical ramus of the mandible and penetrates the capsule of the parotid gland. The facial nerve should recover completely within 2 or 3 hours when the effects of the analgesic solution are wearing off, and there should not be any residual paralysis as it is extremely unlikely that the needle has caused direct trauma to the nerve.

If this complication occurs then the patient must be reassured that recovery will be complete. During the period when the facial paralysis is present, the patient will be unable to close the eyelids on the affected side (*Fig.* 14.10) and hence the cornea must be protected. This may be done by placing drops of sterile paraffin into the eye. The patient should be warned against rubbing the eye or going outside where wind may blow grit into it and, if this is unavoidable, then an eye-shield or eye-pad and bandage should be worn.

Stoy and Gregg (1951) reported a case of facial paralysis which followed an inferior dental nerve block and persisted for 6 weeks, after which there was complete recovery. This patient complained of pain in the ear which supported the conclusion that this paralysis was the result of a vascular reflex causing ischaemia in the region of the stylomastoid foramen through which the facial nerve emerges.

3. Visual complications

These are very rare and difficult to explain. There have been several cases reported of transient amaurosis (i.e., blindness without a demonstrable lesion of the eye) and even permanent blindness following the administration of inferior dental nerve blocks. Although vascular spasm might have accounted

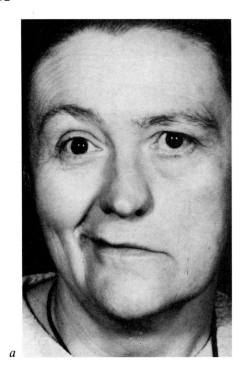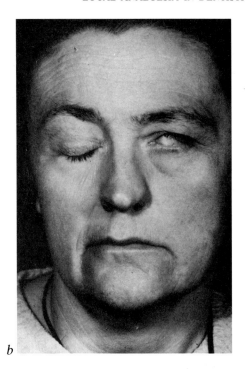

a   *b*

Fig. 14.10. Left facial palsy following an inferior dental injection. The patient is unable to close the eye completely on the affected side.

for some of the cases, it is thought that the most likely explanation is accidental intra-arterial injection of local analgesic solution in patients with uncommon vascular patterns. In these subjects it is presumed that the orbit is supplied either wholly or in part by the middle meningeal branch of the maxillary artery, and this is in part substantiated by the fact that this anomaly has been described in detail in the anatomical literature. No treatment is necessary other than reassurance, as vision usually returns in 10–20 minutes.

Transient squints and double vision have occurred, usually following posterior superior dental or maxillary nerve block injections. These complications have been due to paralysis of the extrinsic ocular muscles and the most likely explanation is that analgesic solution has diffused into the orbit from the pterygopalatine and infratemporal fossae via the inferior orbital fissure. By these routes the solution may affect the oculomotor, trochlear and abducent nerves which innervate the muscles attached to the eyeball. Fortunately these disturbances of

vision pass off within about 3 hours. Another injection which may cause diplopia is the infra-orbital nerve block due to the analgesic entering the orbit.

4. Trismus

Sometimes during the administration of an inferior dental nerve block the needle trauma-tizes the medial pterygoid muscle. This may cause spasm in the muscle resulting in trismus or reduced opening of the mouth. This condition usually resolves within a week and may be helped by local heat applied in the form of hot saline mouthbaths, which are retained at the back of the mouth to provide warmth in the region of the injection.

Another cause of trismus has been described by Killey and Kay (1967), who suggest that with the use of very fine modern disposable needles there is a greater chance of penetrating a small artery. Rupture of the vessel would lead to haematoma formation with subsequent organization of a restricting band of fibrous tissue in the region of the medial pterygoid muscle. This hypothesis accounts for the gradual onset of the trismus over 3 or 4 days and the mechanical locking effect achieved. The condition is relieved by gently prising the mandible open under a general anaesthetic using wide-bladed instruments, such as Featherstone gags, bilaterally in the molar regions. This treatment breaks down the fibrous bands which have been limiting the jaw opening.

Another cause of trismus is infection developing after an injection, usually one given to block the inferior dental nerve. This complication is described later in this chapter.

5. Pain during and after an injection

It is sometimes normal for there to be slight discomfort during or following an injection, but if this soreness is excessive then the reason for this complication should be sought.

a. Due to a chemical irritation: Formerly pain might have arisen from irritation due to the local analgesic solution, but nowadays the drug manufacturers produce them approximately isotonic, almost non-irritant and with a reasonable pH. However, it is interesting to note that where a vasoconstrictor is added to the solution (*Table* 4.1), then the pH is always, of necessity, much lower and therefore more likely to cause pain on injection. If the syringe needle has been kept in a chemical antiseptic such as surgical spirit then contamination of the needle by this may cause a painful injection. It is a good routine to squirt a little analgesic solution through the needle prior to giving the injection. The purpose of this procedure is not only to check that the needle is not blocked, but also to flush away any contaminants within its lumen.

The use of chemical solutions for sterilizing needles is inferior to other methods and there is no justification for it, particularly now that many types of presterilized needle are available.

b. Due to trauma: The use of a blunt needle increases the pain during injection because more force is required and, subsequently, there is increased postinjection discomfort due to the additional trauma. The extremely fine-gauge disposable needles are very liable, if they hit bone, to develop hooked points and thus lacerate the tissues, particularly on being with-

drawn. A sharp needle should be used for every injection and by employing disposable needles this ideal may be readily achieved.

After-pain may arise from trauma to the relatively sensitive periosteum. This layer may be damaged directly by the needle, or distended by a subperiosteal injection in which the analgesic solution separates it from the underlying bone. For this reason the needle should be withdrawn a little before injecting if its point has contacted bone. Normally subperiosteal injections are unnecessary as satisfactory analgesia will be obtained if the solution is deposited external to the intact periosteum.

Pain occurring when the analgesia wears off is frequently due to self-inflicted trauma by the patient. It is very easy to nibble or chew the tissues when they lack sensation because of an injection. This is particularly liable to happen with children and especially when an inferior dental injection of a long-acting analgesic has numbed the lower lip (*Fig.* 14.11). All patients should be warned of this complication.

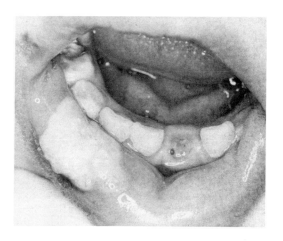

Fig. 14.11. Self-inflicted traumatic ulceration of a child's lower lip following an inferior dental nerve block. (Reproduced by courtesy of Professor G. B. Winter.)

6. Failure to obtain analgesia

Occasionally an injection of local analgesic is completely unsuccessful or analgesia may be partially achieved but inadequate for the proposed treatment. The commonest cause of this complication is an inaccurately given injection in which the solution is not deposited near enough to the nerve. This can be overcome by repeating the injection and taking particular care that the needle is sited correctly in the tissues. Patients vary in size and shape and this is particularly noticeable when giving inferior dental nerve blocks due to the normal variations in the mandible. Another possible cause mentioned previously is accidental intravascular injection in which the solution enters a vessel and is carried away from the nerve via the bloodstream. The complication of incomplete analgesia with the periostitic tooth was discussed in Chapter 7. It appears that in a very few patients, even with accurate injections, it is impossible to obtain complete analgesia and the reason for this is not understood. It is possible that on rare occasions there may be abnormal innervation or the patient has an unusual reaction to the analgesic which renders it ineffective.

7. Infection

If an unsterile needle is used, or if the local analgesic solution is contaminated, then infection may occur. If the injection is superficial, such as an infiltration into the palatal mucosa, then a localized abscess or ulcer may result, whereas infection at the site of an intraosseous injection can lead to osteomyelitis which has also been reported following infiltration injections. When a deep injection is given, the consequences of infection may be serious or even fatal. It may produce a toxaemia which causes the patient to feel unwell, run a high pyrexia, and depending upon the site of infection, have other signs and symptoms such as marked facial swelling, trismus, dysphagia or difficulty in swallowing. A cellulitis may result from spread of the infection in the tissue spaces surrounding the jaws (*Fig.* 14.12).

Infection arising from an inferior dental injection may involve the pterygomandibular space which is bounded laterally by the medial aspect of the vertical ramus of the mandible and medially by the medial pterygoid muscle. Similarly, the lateral pharyngeal and retropharyngeal spaces may be involved and from these infection may pass anteriorly into the submandibular and sublingual spaces, superiorly to the base of the skull, and inferiorly through the posterior mediastinum to the thoracic surface of

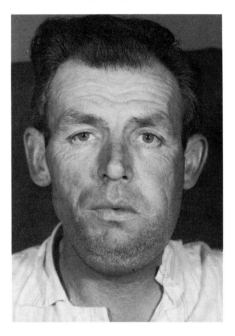

Fig. 14.12. Cellulitis involving the submandibular and sublingual spaces following an inferior dental injection.

the diaphragm. In the neck the lateral pharyngeal spaces extend laterally deep to the carotid sheath, and into the posterior triangles of the neck. In several cases treated by the authors, infection arising from inferior dental injections led to marked trismus and in some of the patients dysphagia was caused by infection tracking medially into the soft palate.

Infection of the cavernous sinus: Infection arising from a posterior superior dental injection may spread via the pterygoid plexus of veins through the foramen ovale, or foramen of Vesalius if it is present, into the cavernous sinus. This is a very serious complication which is often fatal and fortunately rare.

The infraorbital injection may also lead to infection of the cavernous sinus, via the anterior facial vein to the ophthalmic veins which drain from the medial part of the orbit directly into the sinus.

Treatment of infection: Infection arising from a posterior superior dental injection should be treated by administering an antibiotic if there is systemic involvement, and by incision and drainage of pus if there is evidence of abscess formation. If the infection is likely to involve the cavernous sinus then anticoagulants could be given to reduce the risk of thrombosis occurring in the sinus.

8. Hepatitis B

This is a serious complication which may arise following an injection using contaminated instruments. It is due to a virus and may not be recognized as having originated from an injection because the incubation period ranges between 60 and 160 days (mode 6 weeks). Hepatitis B infection is detected by screening for Hepatitis B surface antigen (HBsAg), previously called 'Australia antigen', and is associated with a greater morbidity and mortality than 'infectious hepatitis' due to hepatitis A virus. The increase in incidence of hepatitis B follows the greater use of needles, as in intravenous drug abuse, blood transfusion, needlestick injury and surgery. The infection is usually transmitted parenterally by blood products (as little as 0·0004 ml of infected blood may be enough), by saliva and other routes such as splashes onto mucous membranes.

This infection may go completely unnoticed. Initial symptoms include fever, malaise, nausea, anorexia (loss of appetite), and aching pains in the back and limbs. Clinical jaundice appears a few days later and lasts for 1–4 weeks and patients should rest until this has cleared and the liver is no longer tender. They should abstain from alcohol, at least until the virus has cleared and liver-function tests have become normal, and drugs which are detoxicated by the liver, such as sedatives, should be avoided. For a long time afterwards such patients will be sensitive to sedatives and also drugs used in local anaesthesia, so that the maximum doses that can be employed must be reduced. Over 90 per cent of adult patients will clear the virus with complete recovery, although some will remain depressed for a long time and up to 10 per cent will become chronic carriers with the attendant risks of eventual chronic liver disease, including cirrhosis and liver cancer in up to half of these 'carriers'.

Foley and Gutheim (1965) reported on 15 cases of acute hepatitis following dental procedures, this included three which were fatal. This represented 30 per cent of the total number of cases of hepatitis in one hospital over a 2-year period and recycled needles used for local analgesia were thought to be the probable cause. Another way in which hepatitis B can be transmitted from one patient to another is by the use of the same analgesic cartridge for two patients. This must never be done and partly used cartridges should always be discarded.

9. 'Needlestick' injuries

This is a generic term applied to accidental injuries occurring to dental staff caused by sharp instruments such as probes, root canal instruments and very frequently syringe needles. These injuries are not usually serious unless they arise from instruments contaminated by blood from patients with conditions such as hepatitis B, AIDS or ARC, when specialist advice should be sought. Previous prophylactic vaccination will provide immunity to hepatitis B by producing a high titre of antibody which can be boosted if necessary by a further injection of vaccine, or with immunoglobulin if there has been no previous vaccination. If a 'needlestick' injury occurs when an AIDS or ARC patient is involved then advice from a consultant medical microbiologist is essential.

COMPLICATIONS ASSOCIATED WITH JET INJECTORS

Besides those caused by injection techniques, jet injectors may produce special complications.

The commonest ones reported are splitting of the mobile oral mucosa due to letting the jet injector nozzle move at the time of the injection, and infection arising from unsterile material being fired into the tissues. The risks of these occurring may be minimized by meticulous cleansing of the mucosa and then taking care to hold the injector motionless when injecting. Whenever possible, the site of injection should be on the immobile attached gingiva or mucosa. *Fig.* 14.13 shows the effect of moving a jet injector when firing it on a lamb's tongue. The resulting wound is about 1 cm long and several millimetres deep.

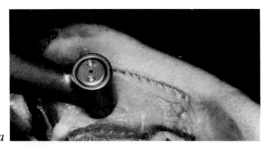

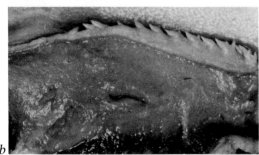

Fig. 14.13. *a, b,* Trauma caused to a lamb's tongue due to not keeping the jet injector still at the time of injection.

REFERENCES AND FURTHER READING

Bishop P. T. (1983) Frequency of accidental intravascular injection of local anaesthetics in children. *Br. Dent. J.* **154,** 76.

Blair G. S. and Meechan J. G. (1985) Local anaesthesia in dental practice. I. A clinical study of a self-aspirating system. *Br. Dent. J.* **159,** 75.

Blaxter P. L. and Britten M. J. A. (1967) Transient amaurosis after mandibular nerve block. *Br. Med. J.* **1,** 681.

Eyre J. and Nally F. (1971) Nasal test for hypersensitivity. *Lancet* **1,** 264.

Foley F. E. and Gutheim R. N. (1965) Serum hepatitis following dental procedures: presentation of 15 cases including 3 fatalities. *Ann. Intern. Med.* **45,** 369.

Fraser-Moodie W. (1958) Recovery of broken needles. *Br. Dent. J.* **105,** 79.

Killey H. C. and Kay L. W. (1967) Trismus following inferior dental nerve block. *Br. Med. J.* **3,** 173.

Killey H. C. and Kay L. W. (1969) *The Prevention of Complications in Dental Surgery.* Edinburgh, Livingstone.

Lederman D. A., Freedman P. D., Kerpel S. M. et al. (1980) An unusual skin reaction following local anesthetic injection. *Oral Surg.* **49,** 28.

Luebke N. H. and Walker J. A. (1978) Discussion of sensitivity to preservatives in anesthetics. *J. Am. Den. Assoc.* **97,** 656.

Meechan J. G., Blair G. S. and McCabe J. F. (1985) Local anaesthesia in dental practice. II. A laboratory investigation of a self-aspirating system. *Br. Dent. J.* **159,** 109.

Rood J. P. (1985) Aspiration in dental local analgesia. In: Derrick D. D. (ed.), *The 1985 Dental Annual.* Wright, Bristol, pp. 152–157.

Standing Dental Advisory Committee (1967) *Emergencies in Dental Practice.* London, HMSO.

Stoy P. J. and Gregg G. (1951) Bell's Palsy following local anaesthesia. *Br. Dent. J.* **91,** 292.

Chapter 15

DENTAL HYPERSENSITIVITY

The problem of a tooth being sensitive to such things as thermal, tactile, osmotic and chemical stimuli is one with which every dental surgeon is familiar. The variety of treatments which have been suggested is all too clear a proof that none has been entirely successful; however, with the introduction of desensitizing toothpastes the problem has come much nearer to a satisfactory solution.

AETIOLOGY

The sensitivity usually takes the form of a sudden sharp pain which can be quite severe. It may be either localized to one or two teeth, or generalized, involving most of the dentition. It is associated with the occurrence of some degree of dentinal exposure due to loss of enamel or cementum, most frequently associated with gingival recession (*Fig.* 15.1). Other causes include the following: abrasion, which can be due to incorrect toothbrushing; attrition, which may lead to exposure of the pulp, es-

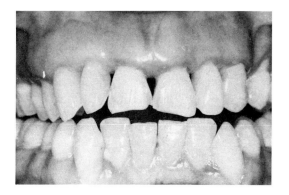

Fig. 15.1. Cervical sensitivity due to gingival recession around the maxillary incisors.

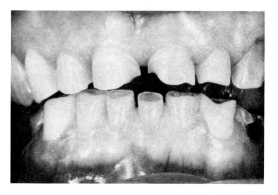

Fig. 15.2. Dentinal sensitivity due to erosion and attrition.

pecially in the lower incisors; surgical exposure of the necks of the teeth by procedures such as gingivectomy; and erosion (*Fig.* 15.2) which is usually idiopathic but may be caused by an acid diet, especially one rich in citrus fruits and 'low-calorie' drinks.

The mode of transmission of pain through the dentine and cementum is not fully understood. The most commonly held theory is that the stimuli are passed down the exposed dentinal tubules by physical or mechanical means to the plexus of nerves lying immediately below the odontoblasts. It has been postulated that the surface tension at the exposed ends of the tubules is altered by the stimuli due to osmotic pressure changes, and that these are then transmitted via the tubules to the odontoblasts, and from these cells to the pulpal nerves. Another theory is that the dentinal fibrils act as nerve fibres by transmitting the stimuli.

Fortunately, few patients suffer from dentinal sensitivity and thus it can be assumed that usually the pulpal tissues are stimulated to lay down a protective calcific barrier which seals off the pulp from painful stimuli.

DIAGNOSIS

The method of treatment of cervical sensitivity depends on whether or not it is localized to one or two teeth. If it is localized then it is important that the affected teeth be identified and that the parts of these which are actually sensitive determined. On occasions the patient can locate the sensitive area quite accurately, often because it is stimulated by toothbrushing. However, if this is not the case, then the surfaces involved can be found by using a probe and running it over the parts of the teeth which one suspects. Another test is the blowing of cold air on to the teeth from an air syringe.

The application of a desensitizing paste such as sodium fluoride causes pain when applied to exposed dentine. Thus if it is rubbed on to the teeth suspected of causing the discomfort one at a time until pain is produced, the sensitive area will be located and treated.

RATIONALE OF TREATMENT

It would seem probable that one or more of three mechanisms are involved in the treatment of dental hypersensitivity:

1. The coagulation of the organic matter in the dentinal tubules which seals them and protects the pulp from irritation.
2. The stimulation of the production of secondary dentine by the pulp.
3. The remineralization of tooth substance. Recent work on this subject has shown that dentine and enamel can undergo remineralization by assimilation of ions from the saliva.

TREATMENT

The following methods of treatment are all of particular use when the patient or the dental surgeon can localize the sensitivity to one or two particular teeth. However, even then it is desirable to reinforce this treatment by prescribing a desensitizing toothpaste.

1. Application of silicones

The commonest method of desensitizing teeth is the covering of the sensitive area with a layer of silicone resin. This is achieved in the case of Tresiolan (manufactured by Espe) by using a mixture of 5 parts of alkyl trialkoxy silane to 1 part of dialkyl dialkoxy silane.

In the presence of humidity, as when applied to the surface of the dentine, a cross-linking polycondensation takes place, and an insoluble silicone resin is formed. This layer of resin is hydrophobic, non-toxic, and produces a considerable amount of desensitization by protecting the tooth against mechanical contact, acids, sweets or cold air.

The teeth to be treated should be cleaned, isolated and dried. The silicone mixture is now applied to the affected area by means of a pledget of cotton-wool held in tweezers and left for 1–2 minutes to solidify. A further application may then be made, this process being repeated two to three times to build up a reasonable thickness of the silicone resin.

One of the main advantages of this form of treatment is that the silicone causes no pain on application, even to very sensitive teeth. Indeed it can be used in cases where it would be impossible to apply sodium fluoride paste satisfactorily without first administering a local analgesic. Further advantages are that it causes no gingival or pulpal irritation and does not discolour tooth tissues.

2. Desensitizing toothpastes

These have superseded all other methods of treatment for generalized cervical sensitivity and are also of great value in treating localized areas of discomfort. They should be used for a period of at least 1–2 months initially and thereafter as and when symptoms recur.

There are two main types:

1. Those containing strontium chloride.
2. Those containing formalin, which is a 40 per cent solution of formaldehyde.

Strontium chloride-based toothpaste

This is marketed under the name of Sensodyne (Stafford-Miller, UK; Block Drug Co., USA) in the UK. The amount of strontium chloride incorporated in the toothpaste is 10 per cent. Many trials have been carried out to test its efficiency and typical results are as follows:

Result	Per cent
Complete relief of symptoms	66
Good relief	16
Fair	11
None	7

By this one can see that only a very small percentage of patients failed to gain benefit from the use of this toothpaste and that it brought complete relief for two-thirds of the people treated. Even repeated treatment by any one of the methods mentioned earlier is unlikely to produce such good results.

Mode of action: The exact method by which this toothpaste acts is unknown; however, it has been shown that strontium chloride deposits considerable amounts of strontium by absorption on powdered bone, dentine or enamel. Thus it would seem likely that the mechanism in reducing or eliminating dentine sensitivity is by absorption of the strontium into the dentine, especially at the ends of the dentinal tubules or within their lumina, with a corresponding blocking of impulses to the plexus of nerves below the odontoblasts. It is also possible that strontium chloride may stimulate secondary dentine formation and thus block sensory impulses at a deeper level.

Advantages and disadvantages: The use of a toothpaste containing strontium chloride has none of the drawbacks encountered by most of the other methods, such as local irritation and tooth discoloration. Its main advantage is that it can be repeatedly and regularly applied without the patient having to attend the dental surgery. Some consider that Sensodyne is too abrasive a toothpaste and should be applied with a finger.

Toothpastes containing formalin
This toothpaste is marketed under the name of Thermodent in the USA and Emoform (Pharmaceutical Manufacturing Co.) in the UK. The compositions are very similar; Thermodent has a 1·4 per cent concentration of formalin and Emoform 1·3 per cent, this being equivalent to 0·5 per cent of formaldehyde.

Several authorities have reported on this material and found complete or good relief in about 75 per cent of cases treated.

In all instances it was found that maximum benefit had been achieved within 3 weeks and that if no improvement had been obtained by this time it was best to either discontinue treatment or support it with local measures. In practice it has been found that if a formalin-containing toothpaste has not been successful by the time the first tube is finished then it is best to change to one incorporating strontium chloride; however, this latter material may take 1–2 months to achieve a satisfactory result.

Mode of action: It is thought that the formaldehyde promotes the coagulation of albumin and organic colloids in the exposed ends of the dentinal tubules, thus gradually desensitizing the surface of the tooth. It should be considered that the formalin may be toxic for the odontoblasts (*see* paragraph 4 below).

3. Application of sodium fluoride paste

The principle of the application of sodium fluoride to the sensitive dentine is that a surface layer of fluoroapatite is deposited which will protect the underlying layers of dentine. It is effective in certain cases, generally requiring two or three applications, but unfortunately the benefit is not permanent. It frequently causes sharp pain at the time of application which usually lasts 30–60 seconds. Do not use acidulated phosphate fluoride (APF) gels because of their acidic properties.

4. Application of formalin

A solution of 15–30 per cent formaldehyde is commonly employed and is thought to act by coagulating the contents of the dentinal tubules so that they become sealed. This technique is not recommended as it tends to kill the odontoblasts.

5. Application of magnesium sulphate

This can be commenced by the dental surgeon, but is more effective if the patient rinses the mouth regularly with a concentrated solution of magnesium sulphate immediately prior to retiring. A toothpaste containing magnesium sulphate can also be prescribed.

Where no response is obtained to any application of medicaments

In these cases, if the area of sensitivity is confined to one or two teeth and is small and easily defined, then the removal of the sensitive dentine and its replacement by a filling with a sedative lining can be considered. Alternatively, where there has been severe occlusal attrition, a full crown may be fitted. However, sometimes the irritation may have persisted for so long that it has caused a chronic pulpitis and in these instances the only possible treatment is devitalization or extraction.

REFERENCES AND FURTHER READING

Smith B. G. N. and Knight J. K. (1984) An index for measuring the wear of teeth. *Br. Dent. J.* **156,** 435.

Smith B. G. N. and Knight J. K. (1984) A comparison of patterns of tooth wear with aetiological factors. *Br. Dent. J.* **157,** 16.

Appendix 1

SUMMARY OF TECHNIQUES OF LOCAL ANALGESIA

The dosages quoted are the average required for a healthy adult using 2 per cent lignocaine with 1 : 80 000 adrenaline.

Site	A. Conservation	B. Extraction	C. Other treatment
Maxillary teeth			
1. Any one incisor	Labial infiltration of 1 ml	As for (A) with palatal infiltration 0·25 ml	For apicectomy the infraorbital nerve block 1·5 ml is recommended with palatal infiltration 0·25–0·5 ml
2. All four incisors	Labial infiltration of 3 ml	As for (A) with long sphenopalatine nerve block 0·25 ml	
3. Canine	Labial infiltration of 1·5 ml	As for (A) with palatal infiltration 0·25 ml	
4. |123	Labial infiltration of 3 ml, or infraorbital nerve block 1·5 ml with labial infiltration of 1 ml over central incisor	As for (A) with palatal infiltration 0·5 ml	
5. Any one premolar	Buccal infiltration of 1 ml	As for (A) with palatal infiltration of 0·25 ml	—
6. Any one molar	Buccal infiltration of 1·5 ml		—
7. Two adjacent molars	Buccal infiltration of 2 ml	As for (A) with greater palatine nerve block 0·5 ml	—
Mandibular teeth			
1. Any one incisor	Labial infiltration of 1 ml	As for (A) with lingual infiltration 0·5 ml	—
2. Canine	Labial infiltration of 1·5 ml, or mental nerve block 1·5 ml		—
3. Premolars	Mental nerve block 1·5 ml, or inferior dental nerve block 1·5 ml	Inferior dental and lingual nerve block 1·5 ml with buccal infiltration 0·5 ml	—
4. 54321 12345	Bilateral mental nerve blocks, total 3 ml	As for (3) *above* for both sides or bilateral mental injections 1·5 ml with lingual infiltrations 1 ml	—
5. Molars	Inferior dental nerve block 1·5 ml	Inferior dental and lingual nerve block 1·5 ml with buccal infiltration 0·5 ml	—
6. Premolars and molars			—
7. 12345678	Inferior dental nerve block with labial infiltration over central incisor 1 ml	As for (5) and (6) *above* with lingual and labial infiltration over central incisor 0·75 ml	—

161

Site	A. Conservation	B. Extraction	C. Other treatment
Very loose teeth			
1. Deciduous	—	Topical analgesia	—
2. Permanent	—	As above, or ethyl chloride spray	—
Oral mucosa			
1. Small superficial layers	Topical analgesia, or jet injection—these may be used prior to taking crown impressions	—	Prior to infiltration injection—as for (A) For local surgery—infiltration analgesia
2. 'Sensitive palate'	—	—	To prevent retching during impression taking or render routine conservation simpler an aerosol spray of analgesic solution can be used or the patient may suck an analgesic lozenge
3. Regions requiring gingivectomy or similar procedures	—	—	Papillary infiltrations, 0·2 ml for each papilla. If root surfaces or adjacent alveolar bone are involved then analgesia of the teeth is required
Difficulties			
1. Where infiltration analgesia fails	Try (a) nerve block, if appropriate, or (b) intraligamentary injection, or (c) intraosseous injection, or (d) general anaesthesia if not contraindicated, or (e) consider sedation only, or (f) consider treatment without any medication, or (g) postpone treatment. The latter methods (e, f or g) should only be used when it is unlikely that the patient will be unduly distressed.		
2. Where a nerve block fails	As for 1 (b), (c), (d), (e) (f) or (g) above.		

Appendix 2

TRADE AND OTHER ALTERNATIVE NAMES FOR DRUGS

Approved name	Trade and other names	Approved name	Trade and other names
Adrenaline	Epinephrine (USP), supra-renin, levorenin	Iproniazid	Marsilid (Roche)
		Isobucaine	Kincaine (Oradent)
Amethocaine	Tetracaine (USNF), Pontocaine, Anethaine (Glaxo)	Isocarboxazid	Marplan (Roche)
		Lignocaine	Lidocaine (USP), Xylocaine (Astra), Xylotox (Pharmaceutical Manufacturing Co.)
Amitriptyline	Domical (Berk), Limbitrol (Roche), Tryptizol (Merck Sharp & Dohme)	Lignocaine hydrochloride	Xylocaine hydrochloride (Astra), Xylotox hydrochloride (Pharmaceutical Manufacturing Co.)
Amitriptyline with perphenazine	Triptafen-DA (Allen & Hanburys)	Lorazepam	Ativan (Wyeth)
Benzocaine	Anaesthesin (Bayer)	Maprotiline hydrochloride	Ludiomil (Ciba)
Bupivacaine	Marcain (Duncan, Flockhart)		
Butanilicaine phosphate	When combined with 1 per cent procaine it is known as Hostacain (Hoechst)	Mebanazine	Formerly Actomol (ICI)
		Mepivacaine hydrochloride	Carbocaine hydrochloride (Pharmaceutical Manufacturing Co.)
Butobarbitone	Soneryl (May & Baker)	Meprylcaine (USNF)	Oracaine (Oradent)
Butriptyline hydrochloride	Evadyne (Ayerst)		
Chlorhexidine gluconate	Hibitane (ICI)	Mianserin hydrochloride	Bolvidon (Organon), Norval (Bencard)
		Midazolam	Hypnovel (Roche)
2-Chloroprocaine	Nesacaine (Pennwalt)	Nialamide	Formerly Niamid (Pfizer)
Cinchocaine	Dibucaine (USNF), Cincainum, Nupercaine (Ciba)	Noradrenaline	Levarterenol (USP), Levophed (Winthrop Laboratories)
Cinchocaine hydrochloride	Dibucaine hydrochloride (USNF)	Nordefrin hydrochloride	Cobefrin
Clomipramine	Anafranil (Geigy)	Nortriptyline	Aventyl (Lilly), Allegron (Dista)
Cresol with soap	Lysol		
Desipramine hydrochloride	Pertofran (Geigy)	Nortriptyline hydrochloride with fluphenazine	Motival (Squibb)
Diazepam	Valium (Roche), Diazemuls (KabiVitrum)	Ornipressin	POR-8 (Sandoz)
Dothiepin	Prothiaden (Boots)	Pargyline	Eutonyl (Abbott)
Doxepin hydrochloride	Sinequan (Pfizer)	Pentazocine	Fortral (Winthrop)
		Pentobarbitone sodium	Sodium pentobarbital (USP), Nembutal (Abbott)
Felypressin	Phelypressine, PLV2, Octapressin (Sandoz)	Pethidine	Meperidine hydrochloride (USP)
Halothane	Fluothane (ICI)		
Hyoscine	Scopolamine	Phenelzine	Nardil (Warner)
Imipramine hydrochloride	Praminil (DDSA Pharmaceuticals) Tofranil (Geigy)	Phenylephrine	Neophryn, Neosynephrine (Winthrop Laboratories)
		Piperocaine	Metycaine (Lilly), Neothesin
Iprindole	Prondol (Wyeth)	Prilocaine	Citanest (Astra)

Approved name	Trade and other names
Procaine hydro-chloride	Novocain (Bayer)
Promethazine hydrochloride	Phenergan (May & Baker)
Propoxycaine	Ravocaine (Cook-Waite)
Protriptyline hydrochloride	Concordin (Merck Sharp & Dohme)
Pyrrocaine	Dynacaine (Graham Chemical Corp.)
Quinalbarbitone sodium	Secobarbital sodium (USP), Seconal sodium (Lilly)
Tranylcypromine	Parnate (Smith Kline & French)
Tranylcypromine and trifluoperazine	Parstelin (Smith Kline & French)
Trimeprazine	Vallergan (May & Baker)
Trimipramine acid maleate	Surmontil (May & Baker)
Vasopressin	Pitressin (Parke, Davis)

Trade and other names	Approved name
Actomol (formerly)	Mebanazine
Allegron	Nortriptyline
Anaesthesin	Benzocaine
Anafranil	Clomipramine
Anethaine	Amethocaine
Aventyl	Nortriptyline
Bolvidon	Mianserin hydrochloride
Cincainum	Cinchocaine
Citanest	Prilocaine
Cobefrin	Nordefrin hydrochloride
Concordin	Protriptyline hydrochloride
Dibucaine (USNF)	Cinchocaine
Dibucaine hydro-chloride (USNF)	Cinchocaine hydrochloride
Domical	Amitriptyline
Dynacaine	Pyrrocaine
Epinephrine (USP)	Adrenaline
Eutonyl	Pargyline
Evadyne	Butriptyline hydro-chloride
Fluothane	Halothane
Fortral	Pentazocine
Hibitane	Chlorhexidine gluconate
Hostacain	Butanilicaine phosphate with 1 per cent procaine
Kincaine	Isobucaine
Levarterenol (USP)	Noradrenaline
Levophed	Noradrenaline
Lidocaine (USP)	Lignocaine
Limbitrol	Amitriptyline
Ludiomil	Maprotiline hydrochloride
Lysol	Cresol with soap
Marcain	Bupivacaine
Marplan	Isocarboxazid
Marsilid	Iproniazid
Meperidine hydro-chloride (USP)	Pethidine

Trade and other names	Approved name
Metycaine	Piperocaine
Motival	Nortriptyline hydrochloride with fluphenazine
Nardil	Phenelzine
Nembutal	Pentobarbitone sodium
Neophryn	Phenylephrine
Neosynephrine	Phenylephrine
Neothesin	Piperocaine
Nesacaine	2-Chloroprocaine
Niamid	Nialamide
Norval	Mianserin hydrochloride
Novocain	Procaine hydrochloride
Nupercaine	Cinchocaine
Octapressin	Felypressin
Oracaine	Meprylcaine (USNF)
Parnate	Tranylcypromine
Parstelin	Tranylcypromine and trifluoperazine
Pertofran	Desipramine hydrochloride
Phelypressine	Felypressin
Phenergan	Promethazine hydrochloride
Pitressin	Vasopressin
PLV 2	Felypressin
Pontocaine	Amethocaine
POR-8	Ornipressin
Praminil	Imipramine hydrochloride
Prondol	Iprindole
Prothiaden	Dothiepin
Ravocaine	Propoxycaine
Scopolamine	Hyoscine
Secobarbital sodium (USP)	Quinalbarbitone sodium
Seconal sodium	Quinalbarbitone sodium
Sinequan	Doxepin hydrochloride
Sodium pento-barbital (USP)	Pentobarbitone sodium
Soneryl	Butobarbitone
Suprarenin	Adrenaline
Surmontil	Trimipramine acid maleate
Tetracaine (USNF)	Amethocaine
Tofranil	Imipramine hydrochloride
Triptafen-DA	Amitriptyline with perphenazine
Tryptizol	Amitriptyline
Valium	Diazepam
Xylocaine	Lignocaine
Xylocaine hydro-chloride	Lignocaine hydrochloride
Xylotox	Lignocaine
Xylotox hydro-chloride	Lignocaine hydrochloride

Abbreviations

DPF—Dental Practitioners' Formulary
BP—British Pharmacopoeia
BPC—British Pharmaceutical Codex
BNF—British National Formulary
USNF—United States National Formulary
USP—United States Pharmacopoeia

Appendix 3

CONVERSION TABLE FOR DOSAGES (Approximations)

Weights: Apothecaries' to Metric

grains	milligrams		grains	milligrams		grains	grams
$\frac{1}{1000}$ =	0·06		$\frac{1}{4}$ =	15·0		20 =	1·3
$\frac{1}{200}$ =	0·3		$\frac{1}{3}$ =	20·0		30 =	2·0
$\frac{1}{150}$ =	0·4		$\frac{1}{2}$ =	30·0		45 =	3·0
$\frac{1}{100}$ =	0·6		$\frac{3}{4}$ =	50·0		60 =	4·0
$\frac{1}{64}$ =	1·0		1 =	60·0		90 =	6·0
$\frac{1}{50}$ =	1·2			grams		120 =	8·0
$\frac{1}{40}$ =	1·5		$1\frac{1}{2}$ =	0·1		150 =	10·0
$\frac{1}{32}$ =	2·0		2 =	0·12		180 =	12·0
$\frac{1}{25}$ =	2·5		3 =	0·2			
$\frac{1}{20}$ =	3·0		4 =	0·25		ounces (avoir)	grams
$\frac{1}{16}$ =	4·0		5 =	0·3		$\frac{1}{2}$ =	15·0
$\frac{1}{12}$ =	5·0		6 =	0·4		1 =	30·0
$\frac{1}{10}$ =	6·0		8 =	0·5		(or nearer, 28·3)	
$\frac{1}{8}$ =	8·0		10 =	0·6			
$\frac{1}{6}$ =	10·0		12 =	0·8		pounds (avoir) 1 =	453·39
$\frac{1}{5}$ =	12·0		15 =	1·0			

Measures: Imperial to Metric (Liquid)

minims	millilitres		minims	millilitres		fluid oz	millilitres
$\frac{1}{2}$ =	0·03		15 =	1·0		1 =	30·0
1 =	0·06		20 =	1·2		2 =	60·0
2 =	0·12		25 =	1·5		4 =	115·0
3 =	0·2		30 =	2·0		5 =	140·0
4 =	0·25		40 =	2·5		6 =	170·0
5 =	0·3		45 =	3·0		8 =	230·0
6 =	0·4		60 =	4·0		10 =	280·0
8 =	0·5		90 =	6·0		(1 pint) 20 =	568·0
10 =	0·6		120 =	7·5		gallon	litres
12 =	0·8		240 =	15·0		1 =	4·546

INDEX